SURVIVING BR
STACEY'

CHAPTER ONE

It was 2008 and I had just moved from Kent to a village in Cambridgeshire, but I was still unsure whether I had done the right thing.
I had previously lived in Ramsgate where I had all my family and friends and my sister living in the same street. I loved it where I lived as I had met so many nice people, who had become my good friends.
I lived alone in Kent with my two Sons my youngest was eleven and my eldest was nineteen, they both meant everything to me.
My house was always full of people but I loved it and my Sons also enjoyed having their friends around as well.
One of my friends lived at the top of my road, he was in his seventies but acted like he was in his twenties, he was still very agile for his age and rode a bicycle everywhere. He became my best friend and he used to come to my house most days to see me. We would sometimes go shopping together or even go out for a quiet drink in the local pub and we used to laugh so much and talk for hours about any and everything. Sometimes I would invite friends around for a party and as my best friend liked rock 'n' roll music I often played it for him, as I to love rock 'n' roll music and my friend and I would be dancing until four in the morning, whilst all the youngsters had already gone home to bed.
One day in 2006 a lady friend called Rose who lived next door to me started talking to me about guys and telling me

I should get out and meet someone new, after all I'd been on my own for about eight years, but I was happy with my life the way it was. But then she suggested going on a date-site and she told me that lots of people do it nowadays, so I took her advice and thought I'd give it a go.
I chatted with quite a few guys and I thought it was quite good fun because I did have a laugh with them, but I wasn't in any rush to meet anyone in person.
After a few months, I did eventually meet a guy who lived locally, but after a few dates I decided he wasn't for me. Then about three months later a guy emailed me and we spoke for a few weeks and then decided to meet.
The guy was a nice-looking guy about six years older than me and when we met we hit it off straight away. The only problem was that he lived in Cambridge which was about a two-hour drive away and because he had to work some weekends, we could only see each other every other weekend.
Just before our first Christmas of seeing each other we'd been together almost two months and he came down to see me. My brother and his wife came around that evening and we all had a nice night. But I later suggested that we all go out somewhere and when I asked my boyfriend if he was up for it he told me I was selfish, I just laughed and so did my brother thinking that he was joking, but then he started shouting at me and things turned nasty. He called me selfish because he'd travelled two hours from Cambridge to see me and he was tired, I said you only had to say that, you didn't have to shout at me, but he wouldn't listen and even my brother and his wife tried to calm the situation down but it didn't stop him.

That night I asked my eldest son to look after my youngest son and just so there was no more arguing I went and stayed the night at my brother's house.

Thinking back now I should have just told my boyfriend to leave, but he couldn't drive as he'd had a drink that night, so in a way I did the right thing by walking away from a bad situation.

The next morning, I arrived home early to find my boyfriend asleep on the sofa and when he woke up he acted as if nothing had happened, but I felt really upset as I couldn't understand what I'd done so wrong. I didn't carry the argument on I let it go but I was still upset and I couldn't stop thinking how badly he'd behaved over nothing.

As Christmas arrived we had a lovely time and things seemed to be going well, but over the months I noticed how quick my boyfriend's mood changed when he had had an alcoholic drink, I then understood why he would have these mood swings. But a lot of the time I tried to ignore him and not argue, but then one day he was in my garden talking across the fence to my neighbour with a drink in his hand and blaring out music, when suddenly I realized my dog had been in the garden. I quickly went outside and told my boyfriend that my dog had pooed on the grass, I also told him to be careful not to stand in it and that I'd go and get a shovel to clear it up. But by the time I'd come back outside to clear it up my boyfriend had stood in it and walked it into my house. He then had the cheek to say to me it's your dog so you had better clean it off my shoe and like a fool I did it. But as I was cleaning it I thought to myself, "*why are you doing this?*", and tears fell from my eyes whist I cleaned his shoe.

I then went to see my sister who only lived down the road from me and I burst into tears, but what I didn't realize was, was that one of her sons was in her house listening to every word I said. I suddenly heard the front door slam and it was then I realized my nephew had gone out and my sister and I had guessed that he had gone to have words with my boyfriend.

A short time later my boyfriend came to my sister's house and apologized to me and I forgave him and went back home.

But over the month's things didn't get any better and even though I'd only see my boyfriend every other week, he would always drink alcohol and start an argument and have me in tears. But in the end, I couldn't take anymore, he came down this certain weekend and started arguing over nothing, so when he did finally go home I text him and told him it was over. I know it was the coward's way out, but it was the easiest way for me as I didn't want any trouble.

But when he saw the text he tried phoning me but I didn't answer him, so he left Cambridge and made his way back down to Kent to my house. He then sat and cried and we both tried to sort things out and as I didn't really want to end things because he wasn't a bad person, he was only bad when he had alcohol, I told him he had to give up drinking and he promised he would.

But the promise didn't last but he did change what he drank, as it was cider that made him moody and then things seemed to get better, until one evening whilst I was having a bath I suddenly heard my music blaring out from downstairs, so I got out of the bath came downstairs and turned it down and I told my boyfriend the neighbours would complain. But he started arguing with me so I started arguing back as I knew I was in the right, but then he called me an awful name (see you next Tuesday), I was shocked and ran upstairs crying, but even after that I still forgave him.

After we'd been together just over a year we talked about me moving up to Cambridgeshire, I had a council home which I didn't want to give up and my boyfriend owned his one bedroom flat. I then put in for a move to a village in Cambridgeshire and went on their waiting list and things seemed to be going well for my boyfriend and I.

As Valentine's day arrived we had a lovely day out together and in the evening, we had friends round, but suddenly things kicked off and my boyfriend's mood changed for the worst, I can't even remember what caused him to start. But as he started shouting at me I decided not to stay quiet I argued back, but it made things a hundred times worse. So I did the one thing I knew he'd hate, I took a puff of my sister in-laws cigarette just to spite him and I gave him something to argue about. He then told me he was going to go and sleep with other women, because if I can have a puff of a cigarette he had every right to go and sleep with someone.

By then I'd really had enough as he'd pushed me to far over the months and as he went to leave I went outside and put a hammer through his car windscreen. Not the best thing I've ever done and I've regretted ever since, because he couldn't go anywhere and the next morning he had a phone call from his Father to say that his Mother had passed away.

I felt awful because his parents also lived in Cambridgeshire and my boyfriend couldn't drive back to be with his Father as he had to have his windscreen mended first. But I always think things are done for a reason and maybe this stopped him driving back home in a shocked state, because he could have quite easily have lost concentration and crashed, not that I'm trying to excuse myself because I'm not.

The next day we both travelled back to Cambridgeshire together and I supported him and his Father throughout their sad time and loss and I even telephoned a housing association asking if they could move me quicker as my boyfriend and his Father needed me with them at that time. Whilst I was in Cambridgeshire awaiting the funeral my sister contacted me to say I had a letter arrive regarding a house in Cambridgeshire, I had to telephone them asap. I was then told I'd got a house in a village in Cambridgeshire and would I be interested in it and of course I was, I viewed the house and excepted it straight away.

When I went back to Ramsgate I had to pack as quick as I could, but everyone was worried about me saying I was rushing things and I shouldn't move away. What made it hard for me was that my eldest son had decided to stay in Ramsgate, but I'd never been away from my boys before, I'd always had them with me. My best friend who I adored immensely begged me not to leave, he told me he'd die if I left, but I said jokingly don't be silly you'll live forever. On the day that I moved my best friend stood in my garden and hugged me, then he pushed me slightly away and walked off up the road, I was devastated because I felt like I'd really hurt him, but I hadn't done it intentionally I loved him with all my heart. But as I said goodbye to family and friends and made my journey to Cambridgeshire, I really wasn't sure I'd made the right decision.

Once in my new house I kept myself busy as I had to get my youngest son who was eleven into a new school and I had the whole house to decorate. My boyfriend was still living in his flat in Cambridge, but he stayed at my house on odd occasions.

When I'd been in my new house about three weeks, I can remember decorating my bathroom and feeling quite ill. I had a heavy period and it was almost as if I was haemorrhaging. I can remember phoning my best friend and telling him how ill I felt and I cried because I felt so weak. After that period, I never had another one, it was as though I'd had about ten in one go and then that was it. But I was only forty-four at the time and I thought surely I'm too young to go through the menopause, so I booked an appointment with a doctor and had a blood test done and they confirmed I'd gone through the change. I never had any other symptoms, no hot flushes, nothing at all, my periods just stopped and that was that.

Over the next few months things seemed to be going well for me, but I really missed my eldest Son and I always thought when I left Ramsgate he would eventually follow, but he didn't and not seeing him as often as I'd have liked broke my heart and I would cry terribly over him.

The first Christmas away from my family was hard because I'd always had my boys with me and my family would always see each other sometime over Christmas. But my eldest son had work commitments so he couldn't get to see me until later in the year.

I kept in- touch with family and friends from Ramsgate and I phoned my best friend all the time, but as Jan 2009 arrived my best friend kept telling me he had pains in his back, he told me it was an old wound that sometimes played him up.

Most days I would speak with him on the phone, but this one day he sounded like he was in a lot of pain, so I told him I was going to phone a doctor to come out to him. He then said you don't have to do that the doctor has just arrived and he then got off the phone. But I wasn't sure whether he was fobbing me off, because he could be quite stubborn and very independent at times, So I phoned my ex next door neighbour Rose and ask her to look up the road and see if there was a doctor's car parked outside my best friend's house and she told me there was, so I knew then he was being honest with me.

A few days later my friend phoned me to tell me he'd been admitted into hospital because of the pain in his back, but a week or so later I couldn't get hold of him on his mobile phone and I started to get quite worried about him. But then rumours started going around the street I used to live in and I had a phone call from my ex next-door neighbour Rose telling me she'd heard that my best friend had passed away, I just collapsed on the floor I couldn't believe. But then I thought I've got to find out for definite for myself as this was just here- say, so I phoned the hospital and they put me through to the ward and told me he was fine and they even let me speak to him on a telephone which was beside him by his bed. I was so relieved I just jumped around the room in my house. But a few weeks after that the phone calls from my best friend stopped and I couldn't find out anything, so as my son had half term from school we both travelled down to Ramsgate and I went straight over to the hospital. I found out my friend had cancer everywhere, but he didn't tell me he'd kept it from me. When he saw me at his bedside he looked at me and said, *"I told you this would happen"*,

I was devastated as I felt like he was blaming me because he was dying, because he had told me before I moved that if I move away he would die.

Those words have never left me but I would never have done anything to hurt my friend as I thought the world of him. That week of half term I spent every day at the hospital and on the Friday night I sat with my best friend all night, his grandson also sat with me, but as Saturday arrived I left the hospital and decided that I couldn't go back to see my friend like that anymore, but instead of going back home to Cambridgeshire I stayed an extra few days at my sisters, as I knew my friend didn't have long to live, so I didn't want to leave until I knew he'd gone and the following Tuesday I had a phone call from his Granddaughter to say he'd passed away and it was then I went back home.

I cried and cried continuously over my best friend and I hadn't cried like that since losing my Dad sixteen years before.

I did go back to Kent for the funeral and even now I still visit his grave and put flowers on for him.

My boyfriend eventually sold his flat and moved in with me on our wedding day, we got married May 2009 and it was one of the hottest days we'd had in a very long time. A few weeks before the wedding my youngest son said to me you do realize you're getting married on the day of the F a cup, but I thought he was joking and I said of course we're not because the F A cup is usually at the beginning of May or the middle, but I was getting married at the end of May. My son then showed me the fixture date and I suddenly burst into fits of laughter, because it was an Everton and Chelsea final and my boyfriend supported Everton and so did my eldest son, but my eldest son supported Everton before I'd met my boyfriend, it was just coincidence they both supported the same team and funny enough my youngest son supported Chelsea.

When I told my boyfriend, he said I'm not getting married then, but I laughed and came up with a solution. Once we were married we came back to the house for food and drinks and I had arranged lots of tables and chairs around the garden and hung bunting around and made it look nice. The men could then go inside and watch the F A cup if they wanted and in the evening, we hired a venue down by the river and we had more food and a disco later in the evening, so it all worked out good in the end.

It was a beautiful day and as I got ready upstairs my friends and family started to arrive from Kent. Once I was ready I was taken to the register office by my boyfriend's Uncle and once there I was taken into a room and asked some security questions, one being what was my Father's name. I had to take a minute to answer as I wasn't expecting the lady registrar to ask me that and it made me quite emotional as it was my big day but my Father wasn't there to give me away. My eldest Son stood in for my Father, as my Father had passed away seventeen years before and my youngest Son was my page boy and stood with my young niece as she was bridesmaid.

As I walked into the room where I was to be married I could see my boyfriend and he started crying as he saw me and it was so relaxed I didn't even feel scared, but I did get the giggles when my boyfriend couldn't get the ring on my finger, I always seem to laugh when I shouldn't.

After the wedding, we went back to the house and then we had a reception in a hired room in a pub down by the river. The D.J played our first song which my husband had chosen, it was by Savage Garden, I Knew I Loved You

Before I Met You. The reason he chose that song was because we knew each other before we met, as we met on the internet date-site. After our first dance, I then danced with my eldest Son, it was a dance for my Father and I chose the song Dance with My Father by Luther Vandross, it seemed the most appropriate song to play and as I loved Luther I think I'd chosen well.

The day went well and everyone had a lovely time and as the night came to an end, my husband and I got a taxi to Ely which was only about five miles away and we stayed in a hotel there which was situated down by the river. We stayed there for two nights, but we were both tired on our wedding night so when we got there we went straight to bed and fell asleep.

But even after that I'd noticed that my husband stopped coming anywhere near me sexually, but I couldn't understand why. When I asked him he just said he was tired and every night when we went to bed he would take a sleeping pill, turn and face away from me and fall asleep. In the end I just accepted it but I still couldn't understand why he didn't want me sexually, but what could I do?.

By this time, I was working at an Environment Agency as a cleaning supervisor, I used to have to lock up and set the alarm as well so there was quite a lot of responsibility involved in the job.

I had now been married about four months and things seemed good.

But then one day I came home from work and got changed and I don't know why I did it but I stood in front of the wardrobe which had mirrors and I checked my breast, it was then I found a lump in my left breast. I called to my husband and got him to feel my right breast and then I told

him to feel my left one. He said, *"it's a bit swollen"*, so I said, *"it's a lump, I've just found it"*.
The thing is I never ever used to feel my breasts for lumps and the one time I did a lump was there, so now I make sure I check myself regularly.
It was a Friday evening so I knew I couldn't get an appointment with a doctor until the following week and what made it even worse was because the following Monday was also bank holiday. So, I had even longer to wait before I could find out anything and be checked over by a doctor.
That weekend felt like a year all I wanted was to get an appointment with a doctor and get it sorted. But once Tuesday arrived I was straight on the phone and I got an appointment quite quickly. The doctor examined me and said it's probably just a cyst, but he'll have to refer me to Addenbrooke's hospital just to be on the safe side. I didn't feel scared because the doctor said it's probably only a cyst, so I thought nothing of it really. Then a few days later I received an appointment to go and have a mammogram at Addenbrooke's hospital, so my Father in-law took me in his car, as it was about a forty-five-minute drive to the hospital and another forty-five minutes back. My husband couldn't take me as he'd just started a new job, so he didn't want to ask for time off so soon, but that was fine by me as I was only having a mammogram.
As I waited patiently in the waiting room there were lots of other ladies in the same position as me, but we all kept our spirits up and chatted to one another.
As I was called in I was asked to confirm my name and address and date of birth and then the nurse stood me by the mammogram machine, I'd never had a mammogram before so the nurse showed me how to position myself and

where to put my arms etc. It wasn't as bad as I thought but I counted in my head to take my mind off it. After I had my mammogram I was asked to wait back in the waiting room and about forty minutes later I was called back in by the nurse.

She then told me that the lump I had wasn't a cyst so I looked at her thinking ok what is it, she then told me not to look so worried as it wasn't cancer, she said if it was cancer we'd tell you, so that was a relief. The nurse then told me that they weren't sure what the lump was so they needed to take a biopsy. I laid on a bed and they gave me an injection to numb the area on my breast and then they took the biopsy, it only took a few seconds and it was all done and I was told to come back in just over a week for the result. I left the hospital feeling relieved because I'd already been told it wasn't cancer, so I assumed it must be fatty tissue or something similar, as they'd also told me it wasn't a cyst. As the days went by I tried not to think about it, but I suppose that was a bit hard for me as I was still curious to know what the lump was. I just continued with my everyday chores including working at the Environment Agency and just had to wait until the day of the results.

CHAPTER TWO

It was Monday 14th September 2009 and I had now received my appointment to go back to Addenbrooke's hospital for my results. My husband came with me that day and it was a nice sunny day and I was feeling fine, not at all nervous.

Before we went to the hospital we stopped off to see my husband's Father and whilst I was there he gave me a gold charm bracelet which was full of charms, which had belonged to his late wife. I thanked him and gave him a hug and a kiss but as I did I noticed my husband didn't look very happy, so I asked him if he was ok and he said yes. But after we left his Father's house my husband told me his Father had no right giving me that bracelet as it had belonged to his Mother and he had bought a lot of the charms on it for her. I said, *but I'm your wife*. He then replied, "*But that charm bracelet should come to me*". I didn't say anything else but I thought how rude he was, did I mean that little to him that he begrudges me wearing his late Mother's bracelet, I couldn't believe what I was hearing.

We soon arrived at the hospital and I sat in the breast Unit in the waiting room when suddenly my name was called by a nurse, I told my husband I'd go in on my own as I knew it was nothing serious. As I walked into a small room there was a male doctor in the room as well, he shook my hand and told me to take a seat. Then he said I've got your results but it's not as simple as we first thought, so I said ok not thinking anything of it. But then he didn't say anything else he just sat looking at me and I was thinking well come on then tell me, but then I looked over at the nurse and she had a serious look upon her face, the penny then dropped, the doctor hadn't said the words but I knew he was trying to tell me I had breast cancer. I was shocked and the first thing I said was that I wanted my husband in here with me.

The nurse left the room to go and get my husband but the doctor and I stayed silent, we never uttered a word to each other. When my husband came into the room I didn't speak to him, I just put out my hand for him to hold and I felt my eyes fill up with tears. The doctor then told me that I would need to have lymph's removed to check the cancer hadn't spread and I would also have to have chemotherapy and radio therapy, but because of the size of the tumour I might even have to have a mastectomy. I was in shock as I had been told that it wasn't cancer just over a week before, so I wasn't expecting it to be this serious.

A brief time later the nurse and doctor left the room to give me some time on my own to get my head around things, but I knew straight away I had to phone my eldest Son. He was at work at the time at Tesco's but I had to tell him first before anyone else found out. I remember how hard it was trying to explain things to him without getting upset, I told him I'd got my results and that I'd got breast cancer, he replied by saying ok. I knew it was a shock for him and I hated having to tell him over the phone, but he was in Ramsgate whilst I was in Cambridge so I had no choice. After I'd told my Son I then phoned my Sister who was also in Ramsgate. I told her the news and she said you'll be fine, you're a strong person and remember our blood group is B Positive, she then said, "*so be positive*" and I never forgot those words. After I'd spoken to my Mother and told her my news, another doctor came into the room to speak with me and he also asked to examine me. He then told me that I had an aggressive cancer and I just panicked.

I can remember that I was lying on a bed and I just felt like I was going to pass out, I was very hot and I just wanted to get up and run out of the hospital, but I knew if I ran I wouldn't be running away from the cancer, it would be running with me. I told the nurse *"that's it then I'm going to die"*, as I remember Caron Keating had had an aggressive cancer and she had sadly died a few years before. I then asked if I could have a wet flannel or something so I could put on my forehead and the nurse went straight out and got me one, just so I could cool myself down.

I then spoke to the doctor explaining that I'd been having pain in my upper back, near my lungs and I was worried that maybe the cancer had spread, so he sent me down for a chest x-ray. As I sat in another waiting room my head was full and the reality of it all was starting to kick in. I can remember crying in the waiting room and I just wanted to get out of there, so I asked my husband to wait there in case my name was called, whilst I went outside for some fresh air. I then phoned my ex next door neighbour Rose and her husband Graham and Graham answered the phone first, so I told him about my results but he couldn't speak he just said, *"I'll go and get Rose"*, he then gave her the phone and I found out later he sat and cried.

After I'd had the chest x-ray I had to wait for the results and it seemed like hours, but everything was fine, it was probably just working in general that had given me back pain.

I then needed to go back to the Breast Unit as the doctor wanted to see me again, but as it was getting late by then I realized my youngest Son would be home from school soon and no one would be there for him, so I phoned a friend who I'd met from my Sons school who had a son the same age as Todd and she said when he gets off the bus which was right near her house, she would keep Todd there until I got home. That was nice of her as that was one less worry for me.

After speaking to the doctor again he gave me an appointment to have the operation on my lymph's and it was in two days time which was quick for NHS patients I thought and I was quite surprised it was happening so soon.

I ended up leaving the hospital about 7pm that evening and by then I just felt totally drained and numb inside.

When I arrived home, I phoned my friend and she walked Todd back to my house and I never said anything straight away to my Son I just asked him how his day had gone at school, but he knew I'd been to hospital that day and he knew it was because I'd found a lump a few weeks before. He then walked over to me and asked if I was ok, I told him no not really and he knew what I meant so he hugged me and a brief time later he went upstairs in his bedroom, so I left him to be on his own for a while and then after some time had passed I decided to go upstairs to see if he was ok. As I sat with him on his bed he said, *"are you going to die?"* I replied by saying *"I hope not"* and I laughed trying to make a joke of it, but I felt like I was being torn up inside, it was awful having to tell my youngest Son something like this, but I had to put a brave face on for him after all he was only twelve years old.

The next day I tried to keep things as normal as possible, my son went to school and my husband went to work and I phoned my manager to explain things to her as I knew I would need time off sick. But that morning my husband came home from work, he had explained everything to his new boss and he told my husband to take the rest of the week off, which I thought was very thoughtful of him. Later that day my husband drove me to the Environment Agency so I could meet with my boss and she was very sympathetic about all that was going on. I was also taken into another room by the receptionist and it was then I was given flowers, chocolates and a get well soon card, I burst into tears as I couldn't believe how kind everyone was being, it was so thoughtful of everyone.

I hadn't slept since the day I'd been diagnosed and I was starting to feel exhausted, but when I went to bed my brain couldn't relax as I had so much going on in my head and it was the nights I hated the most, because in the daytime I could talk to people on social media or phone people, but at night time I felt so alone. My husband would take a sleeping pill and fall asleep and I was left lying awake fearing that the worst was eventually going to happen to me.

As the next day arrived I got myself ready to go to the hospital for the operation on my lymph's and this was one operation I was dreading. I'd had a few operations over the years, including my appendix being removed and a caesarean section from my eldest Son, but I was dreading having my lymph's removed because I was scared of what they were going to find once they'd opened me up.

I remember my husband going to get himself a drink whilst I lay on a bed in the ward and suddenly a nurse looked at me and told me I looked ill, I then explained to her that I'd only found out two days before that I had breast cancer and I explained that I couldn't sleep. She sat and spoke with me for a while and even told me what food I should eat to help me build myself up, everyone was helpful and kind at the hospital.

I had to have my blood taken that day and then I was sent to room to be examined by a nurse, then suddenly she held a long needle and told me she had to inject me with a blue liquid as this would show any cancer that had spread, but it was when she told me I had to have the needle go into my nipple that scared me. I just lay on the bed dead still and closed my eyes, but I was amazed as I never felt a thing apart from a slight scratch, it was nothing like I'd thought it would be.

I was then sent back to the ward and not long after a doctor came to my bedside and asked me to walk down to surgery, I was so scared I cried all the way there, with the doctor walking beside me.

Once I was put out I obviously didn't know anything until I woke up, I remember feeling very tired though. A few hours later the doctor came to see me and explained what they had done, they had taken three lymph nodes from under my arm and I had to come back for the results about twelve days later. They said it didn't look like the cancer had spread but until they had my results back they couldn't be certain.

After a while later I was released from hospital and my husband and I made our way home. But once I was home the pain relief started to wear off and the cut under my arm began to feel quite sore.

Three days later which was Saturday 19th September 2009 I decided I needed to see my eldest Son and the rest of my family and friends in Kent, I knew once I started chemotherapy it would be awkward for me to travel, so it was best to see everyone before starting my treatment.

I arrived at my Sisters house and my Mother and a few friends were already there waiting for me, but as I entered her house I told everyone not to hug me, as I was in a lot of pain through the operation I'd just had having the lymph's removed from under my arm.

After I'd been there a while my Brother arrived and he said he wanted to give me something, it was a bottle of Lourdes water, my Brother had been given two bottles years before from someone when he was a child as he suffered quite bad from asthma.

For those who don't know about the Lourdes water it is a true story about a girl who lived in Lourdes France, her name was Bernadette Soubirous and she was born in Lourdes in 1844.

When Bernadette was fourteen years old she was out with her sister collecting firewood, when she suddenly saw a vision of a lady. Bernadette would often go to the same place and pray in front of the lady and she even told people in the village what the lady was wearing. She wore a white veil and a yellow rose on each foot and the description she was giving was of the virgin Mary, but when officials interviewed her they thought she was simple minded and didn't believe her. But Bernadette kept to her story and kept visiting the same place every day, insisting she was telling the truth. She said the lady told her she was the immaculate conception, but Bernadette didn't know what that meant and it was then that everyone started to believe her story.

One day as she was praying in front of the lady she started digging at the dirt with her bare hands, the villigers couldn't understand why, but as they watched in amazement water appeared and it just kept coming from nowhere. Everyone who had witnessed this miracle knelt and prayed with Bernadette and she was eventually believed and this water became healing water and was known as the Lourdes water

Bernadette eventually became a nun and moved to Nevers France where she died at the age of thirty-five from Tuberculosis of the right knee, she was buried in Nevers, but the town of Lourdes wanted her remains brought back to Lourdes and ten years after her death her body was exhumed, but when the people saw her body it was incorrupt without a blemish. Bernadette was declared a Saint of the Catholic Church by Pope Pius x1 in 1933 and that's where the title St Bernadette came from.

When my Brother gave me this water that meant everything to me, because it was known as Holy water and I still have that bottle of water on a shelf in my living room so I can see it every day.

My eldest Son Adam arrived at my Sister's house later that day as he'd had to work and when I saw him he gently hugged me and I cried. Being away from him was just the worst feeling and not knowing whether I would see him again because of my ill health made it even harder.

I explained to everyone what treatment I had to have in the coming weeks and told them that I would lose my hair through Chemotherapy, but everyone was supportive saying I'd still look lovely with or without hair.

My ex-next door neighbour Rose was also at my Sisters house as she only lived half way up the road, I got on great with her and her husband Graham, they were good friends of mine. But the one person that was missing was my best friend who had passed away seven months before, but maybe that was for the best that he wasn't there, as he'd have been devastated if he'd known I'd got breast cancer, still feels weird that we were so close and we both had cancer the same year though.

I even had another neighbour come to my Sisters house and speak with me, as she'd had a breast operation as well, she showed me her scar but I would never have known if she hadn't told me.

It's quite strange really when you look around at people and their getting on with their everyday lives, but most of them have a story to tell about being ill, but unless they tell you sometimes you just never know. It was surprising how many people spoke to me at the hospital and they looked fine, but inside they were very poorly. I remember talking to a lady whose husband was ill, but when I got talking to her I found out that she had a brain tumour herself but she didn't even look ill.

Whilst at my Sisters I played my wedding DVD to friends that hadn't seen me get married, but as I watched the dance between my eldest Son and I, I just burst into tears, it had got too much for me and I think that's why I got so emotional.

When it was time to leave it was the worst feeling as I didn't know when I would see my family and friends again, or if I ever would. I cried most of the way home but mostly because I had to leave my eldest Son behind, I couldn't bear being without him and I understood that he was twenty years old by then, but to me he was still my baby.

When we arrived home I felt quite empty and what made it worse was because my house was so quiet and I wasn't used to having no one around, but I didn't know many people in the village where I lived, so I didn't have many people to talk too.

I had now started to eat more healthily although I wasn't over weight I was quite thin, but I used to eat any and everything and not always what was good for me. I was told by the nurse to eat plenty of fish as that had lots of protein in it and vegetables such as broccoli were supposed to be an anti-cancerous food. I was even told to buy Manuka Honey as that was supposed to help cure cancer and even though I hate honey I still bought it and unwillingly ate a spoonful a day, sometimes more. I would have eaten dirt from the garden if I thought it would cure me, but no one recommended that to me so I just stuck to the food I was told would make me healthy. I knew I had a long road to recovery ahead of me and I knew I would soon be having a lot of different medicines and chemicals pumped into my body, so I had to eat healthily as I wanted to be strong to survive the next few months.

I was due to start chemotherapy the following Friday, which was only a week and two days after my operation for the lymph's being removed, it all happened very quickly and I'd recommend Addenbrooke's hospital to anyone.

I was quite worried about having Chemotherapy as I'd read and heard so much about the side effects, I was also a bit naive as well as I didn't know how they administered Chemotherapy into someone's body, I thought maybe I had to swallow medicine, I really wasn't sure how it worked.

The week leading up to having Chemotherapy wasn't nice as I couldn't sleep and I seemed to be over the hospital almost every day. It was all very tiring and I felt drained before I'd even started my treatment.

I remember my next-door neighbour who I'd only known about four months, she offered to take me to the hospital one day before Chemotherapy as my husband had to work, he couldn't keep taking time off as he might have lost his job. My neighbour sat with me whilst I was examined by a doctor and I also had an ultra sound scan that day. I was having a clip placed into me which they would attach onto the tumour, it was a bit like a staple. As the nurse positioned the scan so that the doctor could see where the tumour was, he then unwrapped a new long needle from a packet and this had to be pushed into the side of my left breast. The needle didn't seem very sharp and the doctor had trouble piecing my skin to insert the needle and it was quite painful. It was almost like trying to push a blunt knitting needle into a balloon and you knew that the balloon would never pop. The doctor even complained to the nurse that the needle was blunt, but instead of getting a brand-new needle to use, he carried on trying to use the blunt one. I laid so still on the bed counting from one to ten and once I'd reached ten I started counting again in my head, it was the only way I could cope with the pain, it somehow took my mind off things. I could feel tears running down my face, but I just laid still and let the doctor do his job. Then suddenly somehow, I felt a pop where the needle had gone in and I made a slight noise as it hurt a bit, but at last he'd finally managed to piece my skin and get the needle inside of me. He then placed the clip onto the tumour and once that was done the nurse cleaned me up as there was blood all over my breast. It must have taken the doctor almost an hour to get that needle in me and I had to just lay there and injure the pain. My neighbour by this time was in tears and I asked her what was wrong. She replied by saying she couldn't believe how brave I was as I didn't move or make a noise apart from when the needle pieced my skin, I just smiled at her and said what other choice did I have.

The reason I had to have a clip placed onto the tumour was because once I started Chemotherapy the tumour would shrink and if it shrunk to much they wouldn't be able to see where it was on the scan and they needed to know its exact position. Now that the clip was in place if the Chemotherapy shrunk the tumour and I had an ultra sound scan, they could find it easily by seeing where the clip was. Once I was up and dressed my neighbour and I went to the café at the hospital and had a hot drink and a cake and I know cakes aren't good for you but I think I'd earnt that by what I'd just been through.

We sat and talked for a while and then we made our way home.

My breast was a bit sore but nothing I couldn't cope with, I was more worried about under my arm where I'd had the lymph's removed. It had swollen up and I had a huge lump under my arm that looked like it was full of fluid, it was so painful and I had trouble when I went to bed as I couldn't lay on that side and even if I tried to turn onto my right side, it was the most painful thing I'd ever had. I did mention it to the doctor at the hospital but I was told that unfortunately it happens sometimes, so in other words I just had to put up with it. I've had a few operations in my life, but I've got to admit having my lymph's taken out has been the most painful operation I've had to date, but I'm not saying that's the same for everyone as everyone is different.

A few days later I was back over the hospital as I had to be examined by the doctor again and be weighed and have a blood test taken. It was the day before I had to start my Chemotherapy and apparently, everyone has to have a blood test before being administered Chemo, just in case there is something wrong with their blood.

My Father in-law took me to hospital that day and although he was eighty-seven years old he still drove his car and was quite spritely for his age. We got on well and I was company for him as he was now on his own since losing his wife. He was quite a funny guy and always made me laugh and we'd sit and talk for hours. I often invited him around for Sunday dinner as I thought it would be nice for him to get out of his house and be somewhere different for a change. I could tell he was lonely but he did keep himself busy with his inventions that he made from home. He was a bit like Del Boy from Only Fools and Horses, he always thought he'd end up being a millionaire, but unlike Del Boy that never happened. But all the while he had inventions to make it kept him going and he was happy.

CHAPTER THREE

It was now the day I'd been dreading the day I started my Chemotherapy and I wasn't looking forward to going to hospital one little bit. My husband had taken the day off to be with me that day and things were good between us since I'd been diagnosed with breast cancer. He hadn't drunk any alcohol so that made a lot of difference, as we got on well when he didn't drink. When I drank, I used to laugh a lot and be happy, but it was the other way around for my husband, it turned him nasty and although he never hit me his verbal abuse was just as bad.
As I arrived at the hospital I sat in Oncology and waited for my name to be called and I've got to admit I was scared.
As I sat there I looked at the hundreds of people around me, some with head scarves on that had already lost their hair and others that had wigs on or hats. But everyone seemed happy and they were laughing and joking with each other, but I couldn't understand why. I was mortified at the thought of having Chemotherapy and I just sat next to my husband and cried.
I waited ages before my name was called and then I was taken into a room by a nurse to have my blood pressure taken. I then asked her why everyone was laughing, as I felt distraught at that time and she told me that in time I would be just like them, but I couldn't see that and I told her I don't think so. But she said to me you will be laughing in a few weeks, but I still didn't believe her.
I was also given tablets to take and some I had to take before Chemotherapy, some after, some were steroids, some were sickness tablets and so on. There were a lot of

tablets I had to remember to take, I had a carrier bag full of boxes of all kinds of tablets.

After having my blood pressure taken I sat back down in the waiting room and it seemed to take ages before I was finally called in to have my first Chemotherapy.

I had been told that I had to have six courses of Chemotherapy, one every three weeks and my hair would start to fall out on the second or third lot of chemo.

I was taken into the room where lots of other patients were also having Chemotherapy and I was asked to sit in a chair. The nurse then explained to me how the Chemotherapy would be administered, it would be put through a drip in my right hand. But for some reason which I don't know why, once you have breast cancer you always must have blood tests and I chemotherapy inserted in the opposite side of where the cancer is situated.

I was told that firstly I would be put on a drip with a wash going through me, then I would have the Chemotherapy dripped into me and then I'd have a drip with wash again at the end. It all looked the same it was a bag of clear liquid for the wash and Chemotherapy.

As I sat there whilst the nurse put a cannula into my hand I was feeling nervous, but then I looked around me and I saw all these other people going through the same thing and I thought if they can do it then so can I.

The wash took about twenty minutes to pump into my body and then I had to have the chemo. I felt fine at first but after a few minutes or so I started to feel tight chested and I started to panic, so my husband called the nurse over and she lowered the amount that flowed into my body. It took a bit longer for the drip to go into me but I felt fine after that.

After about thirty minutes the Chemotherapy bag was empty, so the nurse gave me another drip with a wash in it, it kind of flushes the Chemotherapy through your body. Then after about another twenty minutes I was all done, but I wasn't allowed to leave straight away, I was made to have something to eat and drink and it was all provided by the hospital.

I then left the hospital with my husband and I didn't have to go back for another three days, as on the following Monday I had to go back to find out my results from having my lymph's removed, they would then tell me whether the cancer had spread to my lymph's.

When I got home my husband cooked me a dinner and gave me all the vegetables I needed to make me healthy again and things were good between him and I once more and where I had doubts over whether he cared for me, now the way he was behaving towards me, I was certain that he did care.

The next day which was a Saturday I felt fine so we went to Cambridge together and we even had a meal out at lunchtime, Todd my Son also came with us and we had a wonderful day. I felt good because I'd now had my first Chemotherapy and I felt like I'd worried over nothing.

I loved walking around Cambridge it's a beautiful City and there is so much to see, it was much better than the village that I lived in as it seemed full of life, not quiet and boring like where I lived. I've always been a town person where I could go to the shops when I wanted, but where I lived I felt a bit trapped as I didn't drive and the buses only came every two hours. Everything was so far out and I hardly knew anyone and I felt quite lonely at times.

I know a lot of people love the quiet life but I'm not one of those people, the louder the better it is for me. I love the countryside and the village I lived in was very pretty and where I used to take my dog for walks was beautiful as I could see for miles and the view was breath-taking. But it's not all about trees as there is so much more to life, seeing a tree isn't going to speak to me or help me when I'm feeling low, I needed friends around me which I didn't have.

I had now gone on social media which I'd never done before, but it was my own way of interacting with people, because apart from when I went to hospital I hardly saw anyone. My husband was at work all week and my Son Todd was at school, so I was left totally on my own and I was beginning to hate it where I lived.

It was now Sunday two days since having my Chemo and I was beginning to feel quite ill, it felt like my head was going to explode and I felt hot. I just wanted to lay down and sleep as I had no energy in me and I couldn't bear any loud noises around me. This was just the start of me feeling ill but it got a lot worse over time.

I can remember going to bed feeling shattered but I couldn't sleep through fear that I was going to die and it was real scary because in the middle of the night I had no one to turn too, my husband had taken a sleeping pill so he was out to the world and everyone I knew would be in bed as it was late, but it was then that I needed someone with me. I couldn't bear lying in bed in the dark as it scared me, so I used to get up and go downstairs and put the television on and lay on the sofa watching TV until I fell asleep. My living room was my comfort zone and it was where I felt safe.

As morning arrived it was the day I had to go back to the hospital to find out my results from my lymph gland operation, but I felt too ill to travel all the way to

Cambridge. The Chemo had kicked in quite bad and I felt like I just wanted to collapse and die. I phoned the hospital and spoke to a young nurse there that I had got to know quite well and she told me that they had my results and it was all clear, so I didn't have to go to hospital after all. I was also told that I wouldn't have to have a mastectomy like they'd originally thought and I was over the moon as I was scared that the cancer may have spread to my lymph glands and once she told me I was clear I just burst into tears. That was such good news and not the news I was expecting, I think when anyone is ill we always expect the worst, but on this occasion, it was the best news I could have asked for and it was one less worry for me.

As I lay on the sofa feeling so ill I cried because I thought *"is this it, is this the life I've got to look forward to"*.

At that time, I didn't know whether I was going to live or die and feeling that ill didn't help, because I felt like this was the beginning of the end.

I slept on the sofa in the daytime and I was totally alone, it was a real scary time, but in the evenings my husband would come home from work and my Son would come home from school and I then had a bit of company.

I hated my Son seeing me so ill it's not what a child of his age should have to see, but he was brilliant and was there for me whenever he could be.

I used to have to force food inside of me because I knew I needed to build myself up, I didn't admit it at the time but I was too thin and I needed to put on a bit of weight, but when I was ill I didn't want to eat but I knew I had to.

I was ill for about three days and then once I was feeling better I had to go straight back over to the hospital for more appointments.

My Father-in-law took me for a scan and I remember I had to lay on the bed face down with my head through a hole and with my breasts peeking through a separate hole and I had to put my arms as high as my head which was quite uncomfortable because the cut under my arm from my operation still hurt, but that was how I was asked to lay so I had no choice but to put up with it. I had to lay like that for about thirty minutes and as I lay there I remember my nose started to run because I was lying face down, but I couldn't do anything about it as I had been told not to move, but when they did finally let me get up off the bed, my nose had dripped everywhere, it was very embarrassing at the time although I can laugh about it now.

My Father in-law and I always went to the café after I'd seen the doctor and we'd have a hot drink and a cake and I think he enjoyed his time with me, it got him out of his house and I was company for him and we got on extremely well.

The week after having my first Chemotherapy my house was empty as my husband was at work and Todd my Son was at school and I suddenly started having bad pains in the top of my back, it felt like indigestion, but I'd never had it in my back before. It was so painful in the end I was crying, but I had no one to help me. I couldn't phone my husband as he was at work and he hadn't been at that job long, so I just had to get on with it. As the time went on the pain seemed to be getting worse and I then remembered that I had my next-door neighbours phone number on my phone, I didn't know her extremely well but I took a chance and phoned her hoping she wasn't at work. Although she had bought the house next to me she wasn't living in it, her husband was doing it up to let out, but they had another house the other side of the village to me which they lived in. She answered the phone and I explained to her what the problem was and a brief time later she drove to my house and then she telephoned the doctor who came out to me a while later. I was in a lot of pain and I told the doctor I thought it was indigestion, but he wasn't so sure so he called for an ambulance. By this time my temperature had gone quite high, but I think that was because I was in so much pain.

My Son then arrived home from school and I explained to him what was happening and he was there when the ambulance arrived. One of the guys put me on a heart monitor as they thought I could be having a heart attack, even though I had told them I thought it was indigestion. But saying that my Father had said that to me twenty-one years before, as he had pains in his back and chest, but it turned out that he had had a heart attack and then he had a second one five years later which killed him. So, in a way the ambulance guys did the right thing as they weren't sure what was wrong.

A brief time later they decided to take me to hospital, I had to travel for forty-five minutes to Addenbrooke's again, but I knew they would soon find out what was wrong with me once I was there.

My Son travelled in the ambulance with me and I text my husband explaining to him I was being taken to hospital. Some of the neighbours came out of their houses as I was carried into the ambulance, they were all friendly neighbours and just concerned about my wellbeing.

One of the ambulance guys sat in the back of the ambulance with me and he was a nice guy, real friendly and he spoke to me all the way to hospital trying to put my mind at ease, I wish I'd taken his name now so I could thank him because he did an amazing job and he was so kind and helpful.

When I arrived at the hospital I was taken to a room on my own and my Son sat with me. Then a brief time later a doctor came in the room to speak with me, so I explained to him what was wrong, I also told him that I had recently started Chemotherapy. He took my temperature and blood pressure and I was again put on a heart monitor, I also had to have blood taken so they could check my blood count.

I had been at the hospital about an hour when my husband arrived, so I explained to him what was going on and I told him they were trying to find out what caused me to have severe pains in my upper back, but by this time the pain had gone so I was feeling a lot better. I was in the hospital hours waiting for someone to come and tell me what was going on and when a doctor did finally come to see me, I was told I was going to be taken to another ward. When I got there I just froze as I was again in a room on my own, but it wasn't like the first room as I knew that I was there as I'd just been brought in, this room was like a proper patient room where patients stayed overnight. The room reminded me of when my best friend was in hospital and I knew he never came out, he died in that room. I panicked because I thought I'd been brought to that room to die and I told my husband I'm not staying here over night, but he told me I'd have to if they wanted to keep me in.

Having cancer and the treatment was all new to me so anything out of my comfort zone frightened me, as I didn't know what to expect or whether I was dying or not.

The nurse then told me my temperature was up so I had to drink plenty of fluids, she also told me my white blood count was low, so they were a bit concerned about that as well.

As I lay in bed I started to get quite bored and all I wanted to do was get of the hospital and go home. I was also worried about my Son as it was getting late and he had to be up early for school the next day.

Just after midnight I was told my temperature had dropped and my heart was fine, the pain had been caused through indigestion but from the side effects of Chemotherapy and I was now allowed home. I was also given some indigestion tablets to take as and when needed and even to this day I still must take them, as I've never stopped getting that pain since having Chemo, but I don't get the pain everyday but I do get it at least four times a week. My Son must sometimes wind me like a baby just to dislodge the trapped wind and I can see why babies cry when they have wind because it is extremely painful.

The nurses wouldn't let me walk out of the hospital they took me out in a wheel chair and my husband had to drive his car to the entrance of the hospital and then I could get in the car. Everyone was nice to me at the hospital but I just panicked as usual being in that room, but I was glad to be finally going home.

It was after one in the morning before we eventually got home, so I let my Son have the next day off school as he was still tired. I did contact the school to let them know and they were very understanding so everything was fine. It was nice having my Son home with me as it did get lonely being on my own and he was great company.

Once the following week had arrived I felt a lot better in myself, but I had noticed how out of breath I'd got since having Chemo, I'd walk so far and then I'd have to stop, I felt old suddenly.

My Father in-law was due to take me to hospital the next day, not to see a doctor I was to have a treat. I was to be given a bag full of expensive makeup and perfumes, but I had to go to the hospital to collect it. It was a way of making cancer patients feel special, as it wasn't nice at all what we were all going through. I was also going to meet up with other cancer patients and be shown how to put my make-up on professionally.

As I was watching television the night before I sat twiddling my hair when suddenly it fell out, I wasn't sure if it was falling out due to the Chemo or whether it was just coincidence, so I twiddled the other side of my hair and the same thing happened. I then called to my husband who was upstairs and I shouted that my hair was falling out, he then said *"whatever"*. I went upstairs and showed him and then I combed my hair and I had a carrier bag full of lose hair where it had fallen out. I was quite shocked as I had been told that on the second or third Chemo my hair would start falling out, but I'd only had one course of Chemo and it had only been a week and a half since the first course and yet my hair was falling out already. I had bald patches all over my head so I knew if I went out I'd have to wear a hat as it looked awful. But then I remembered that Addenbrooke's hospital had their own hairdressers, so I phoned them the next day and told them I was due to come over to collect some make-up, so they managed to book me in that same day.

My Father in-law drove me to the hospital and I went straight to the hairdressers and I showed the hairdresser the state of my hair, I also asked her to shave it off there and then. I had long hair so it was an important thing for me to take such drastic action, but I knew I couldn't go out and let people see my hair with bald patches in it, so I closed my eyes and the hairdresser shaved it all off.

I didn't feel as bad as I thought I would, I think I was more worried about it growing back and that I'd have to have short hair for a while, because I hated short hair on me it just doesn't suit me.

I put my hat back on and looked at my Father in-law, he just smiled at me and nodded just to let me know it was ok. I was so lucky I had him as a Father in-law, but he was also a friend and he meant a lot to me.

We then went to collect my make-up and I had to go to a room in the hospital and there were ladies already there seated around a table. I sat down with them and we were each given a vanity bag with lots of make-up inside it and it wasn't cheap make-up it was Max Factor, Chanel, Revlon etc and perfumes as well. We then sat together whilst a lady showed us how to put on our make-up and it was quite a fun day, it felt nice mixing with people again as I'd missed the company of my friends back in Kent and it made us as cancer patients forget that we were ill, for a while anyway.

My Father in-law sat in a chair behind me just watching us ladies laughing and enjoying ourselves and I got to admit he was very patient as he must have been bored really.

After that we all left the room and my Father in-law told me how beautiful I looked and although I had not long had my hair shaved that day, I didn't feel as bad as I thought I would.

When I arrived home, I showed my Son my head, (not my hair ha ha) and he smiled and told me I was now a slap head, that made me laugh the cheeky thing.

My husband came home from work late that day and I was beginning to get quite worried, but then there was a knock at the door which I thought odd, as no one used to come to my house very often since I'd moved to a village. I got up from the sofa and opened the door and my husband was standing there with his hair cropped. He used to have it spiked but he'd had it cropped short out of support for me, well that's what he told me. I was really pleased he'd done that for me it meant a lot.

The next day which was a Friday was the same old thing for me, sitting on my own bored out of my head. I still did my chores such as washing housework etc, but when vacuuming I could only do one room and then I'd have to sit down for a few minutes before continuing the next room. The chemo had made me very out of breath, it felt like I'd aged thirty years overnight.

I used to phone my Father in-law every day to make sure he was ok and we'd have long chats which helped break my day up. But I missed having my friends around from Kent and I had started to feel lonely and secluded, but there was nothing I could do about it.

As the weekend arrived I went shopping for food with my husband and Son, but I got tired very quickly and as soon as I got home I had to lie down on the sofa. My husband told me he wanted to go to the pub to have a drink and yet it was early afternoon, I didn't say anything I just let him go but I thought he was a bit mean leaving me on my own, knowing I'd been on my own most of the week, well apart from when I had hospital.

I sat and cried that day as I felt like I had no one, but then my youngest Son Todd sent me a text saying, *"don't cry Mum everything will be ok"*.

He had been watching me through the gap in the door and I didn't realize, he then came into the room and hugged me and I cried even more.

When I was first told I had to have Chemotherapy, the doctor said I might get really bad tempered, but I went the other way I used to get emotional quickly and cry a lot. My Son and I sat and watched the Lion King together that day, that was my favourite Disney film and it felt nice snuggled up with my Son with a duvet over us.

When my husband finally returned many hours later he was drunk as a skunk and he started telling me how people had reacted to him having his hair cropped. He said to everyone that he fancied a change of image, but he never once mentioned that I was ill to anyone. I didn't say too much to him because I knew if I said the wrong thing he'd start an argument and I just couldn't be bothered to argue back. My husband got something to eat and then went upstairs and laid on the bed and watch television from upstairs, he didn't sit with me like my Son had earlier.

A brief time later I went up to bed but my husband was fast asleep and snoring loudly, he was drunk and had taken a sleeping pill so there was no way I would be able to wake him, so I went back downstairs and slept on the sofa. The next day my husband was hungover so he spent the entire day in bed and that was my not so fun weekend over with.

CHAPTER FOUR

On the Monday, the very next day, my Father in-law came to see me, he lived about thirty minutes' drive away. He would often come to visit me to give me a bit of company and it also gave him company too.
He'd stay for quite a few hours and sometimes he would stay longer as I'd cook him dinner and we'd chat for ages. It was the most company I got because I hardly saw anyone throughout the day, I was extremely lonely and I was starting to get depressed.
As the week went on I was dreading it as my second Chemotherapy was due at the end of the week. I had to go to hospital the day before Chemo to have a blood test and then on the day of my Chemo I had to be weighed and have my blood pressure taken before having Chemo.
My Father in-law took me both days. He was so good, he was amazing and if it hadn't been for him helping me, I don't think I'd be here today to tell my story.
I made friends with one lady at the hospital as we'd been diagnosed with breast cancer around the same time, we had something in common so we had a lot to talk about. She was quite a bit older than me but we got on well.
I remember talking to her one day when we were both waiting to be examined at the Breast Unit in the hospital, I said to her if we get to tired and don't want to go out, we could always use the excuse, "sorry *I've got to wash my head*" ha ha. That made her laugh and even a guy sitting near us over heard what I'd said and he smiled at us as well. Although we were going through an horrific time, we never lost our sense of humour.
It's surprising how many people are going through cancer treatment and you don't even know, because some people

don't always lose their hair and even if they did they'd wear a wig and sometimes you wouldn't even know.

I went to the hospital one day to look at the wigs and they were free to cancer patients. I chose one but I only wore it once, but I had seen a nice one online which I liked, it was more me. I wore it to Kent one day as I visited my family and it was long so I tied it up in a long lose pony-tail and put a hat on top.

When I arrived at my Sisters if I hadn't told them I'd already lost my hair they wouldn't have known, as the wig looked like my own hair that I'd had.

After being there a while I pulled the hat and wig off so everyone could see what I looked like with no hair and everyone told me it suited me, I wasn't so sure though.

I never wore a wig again I just used to wear hats as I felt more comfortable in them and I had some nice hats in the end.

As I sat waiting for my second course of Chemotherapy the nurse put the cannula into my right hand and I didn't like to look as it went in, so I used to turn my head away. But this one day I saw a lady who was obviously having Chemo as well sitting opposite me, but I could see a tube coming out from her chest. I never said anything but I wasn't sure what cancer she had, as hers was being administered differently to mine. It surprised me though because after I'd had my first course of Chemo, I thought everyone had it administered in their hand, but obviously not.

The second time I had Chemo I was fine I didn't cry, I was laughing and joking with people just like the nurse had told me I would be a few weeks before.

When you're first diagnosed it's such a scary feeling and you don't know how to escape from it, but then again there is no escape. I sometimes felt like the fear of having cancer was worse than the treatment.

My Father in-law sat with me whilst I had my Chemotherapy, but it must have been hard for him to watch as it had been less than two years since his wife passed away from Leukaemia. But he was a good-hearted man and he never once complained about taking me to hospital and yet I had lots of appointments every week, the only time I didn't have to go to hospital was the week after I'd had Chemotherapy, as that was my ill time.

The more courses of Chemotherapy I had the weaker I felt and I'd even started to hallucinate because of it.

One day I was lying in bed and I could see thousands of small bouncy balls all around me coming down from the sky and I could see my nephew Billy from a distance, so I called to him and he walked towards me and hugged me. But I suppose Chemo effects everyone differently. I had quite a strong Chemotherapy and it did make me very ill, it was a trial one and the doctors asked if they could use it on me. I didn't refuse because I just wanted to be made better, I think if I remember rightly it was called the Artemis Trial.

After having my second Chemo my Father in-law and I made our way to the café once more, so we could have our favourite Mars Bar cake, they were delicious and we always looked forward to them.

I had now started to put a bit more weight on and no not through eating to many cakes, I only ate them now and again. I put weight on through all the tablets I was taking, I was on quite a lot of steroids as well. I really don't know how I remembered to take all those tablets, because I had boxes of them and I'd placed them in sections on my dressing table and somehow, I knew exactly which ones to take on which days.

The next day which was Saturday my husband and I went food shopping again, it was the highlight of my week as I didn't get to do much else, I didn't like going out on my own much as I sometimes felt quite weak.

Every time we went food shopping my husband would place all his food in a separate basket and only pay for his own food, I had to buy my own food for myself and my Son. I even had to pay for all my Son's school uniform and if he needed any new clothes or shoes I'd have to buy them as well, my husband never once contributed. But I'd buy joints of meat or chicken and mince and if I did a roast dinner or a shepherd's pie I'd cook it for all of us as a family and even invite my Father in-law for dinner. But my husband never shared his food, what he bought was his and god help my Son if he helped himself to one of my husband's biscuits, he'd go mad.

After we'd got home from shopping my husband decided to go to the pub yet again, but this time I begged him not to go as I didn't want to be on my own and his answer to that was *"I'm bored with watching you sleep"*. I couldn't believe what I was hearing. How could he be so insensitive knowing what I was going through? I just told him to go in the end as I felt I'd be better off being on my own, as he wasn't any help to me. I still had my Son Todd at home with me and he had become my rock, he was so supportive to me and yet he was still so young, bless him.

When my husband eventually came home from the pub he was drunk again and he tried to start an argument, but I just ignored him as I wasn't well enough to argue with him. I then sat by myself thinking, *"Is this what my life has become"*?

I even thought, *why on earth did he have his hair cropped*? Because it wasn't really for my benefit, thinking about it now I think he just wanted the attention on him.

"*What kind of marriage was I in*"? I was with a man who got drunk every weekend, never came near me sexually and never wanted to go anywhere with me apart from food shopping. All he wanted to do was go to the pub when he had any free time.

I often spoke to my Father in-law and confided in him about his Son's behaviour, after all I didn't have anyone else much to talk to and I was also beginning to think that all my family and friends in Kent were right, maybe I was wrong to have moved away with him.

As I became quite ill the next day my husband was still argumentative, so I said to him, "*please don't start I really don't feel well*" he then said to me, "*Oh yes I forgot you've got cancer and its always about you*". I couldn't believe anyone could be that crawl. I then said to him "*Well I'm sorry for being ill*".

This felt like the beginning of the end for us, as I was beginning to despise him.

About ten days later I decided to go to Ramsgate Kent for a week and take Todd my Son with me as it was half-term, I felt like I needed the break away, so I stayed at my Sister's house.

I did let the hospital know that I was going away and they were fine, I just had more appointments to attend once I got back to Cambridgeshire.

Whilst in Ramsgate I met up with friends I hadn't seen for ages and I had a lovely time, it was so nice being around everyone again. I even met up with my eldest Son Adam on his day off and we went out for breakfast and I saw him some evenings whilst I was in Kent as well.

Although I wasn't on my ill time I still had days where I felt totally drained and would often feel sick.

I remember when I was back in Cambridgeshire I got up early one morning to do my Son's pack lunch for school and as I was buttering the bread I just felt so ill, I called to my husband to come downstairs as he hadn't left for work at that time and I just laid down on the kitchen floor. It felt nice because the floor was cold and I felt very hot. I told my husband to just leave me where I was and I asked him to finish off making my Son's pack lunch.

My dog must have sensed that I was ill because normally if I laid on the floor he'd have jumped all over me, but this day he didn't he just laid in his bed looking at me.

One day whilst I was laying down on the sofa my dog climbed up behind me and started licking my bald head, it's as if he knew I was ill and he was trying to help me. It's funny how animals sense things, but they do.

I had a thermometer at home which a neighbour had kindly bought me, because I had to keep a check of my temperature and if it got to high I had to phone a doctor immediately.

I still had to have lots of appointments at the hospital and I had to have more scans, I didn't always have to lay face down though but on some occasions, I had to have a red liquid put into me before the scan and later when I'd left the hospital if I peed it came out red like the liquid.

Before my third course of Chemotherapy I was booked in to have an ultra sound scan, that's the type of scan you have when you're pregnant. As they scanned me they found where the clip was situated on the tumour, but the doctor was surprised how quickly my tumour had shrunk. I was over the moon as the Chemo was working, this was just the best news ever.

Leading up to my third Chemo I was dreading it, not because I was worried about having it done, I was more worried about how my husband was going to behave towards me on my sick time. I'd even confided in my family about his behaviour and they weren't happy with him at all.

The day before my third Chemo I had to see the doctor at the hospital and she explained to me that after this course of Chemotherapy they would be changing it to a different Chemo, she also said it would probably make me feel even more ill. I thought to myself *"Great that's all I need"*. But I knew I had to have it to make me better again.

I also had to go to the Breast Unit that day to speak with a nurse, it was then I was asked if I'd take part in a survey, I didn't really know much about it but I still agreed to take part. I was given an envelope with lots of paperwork inside, but I didn't look through it all straight away, I took it home and put it to one side.

The next day I had my third course of Chemotherapy and in a way I was pleased because I knew I was half way through my treatment.

I sat talking to a young guy who was having Chemotherapy next to me and I said to him, *"It's awful isn't it?"* he agreed and said, *"You can't explain what It's like to anyone, they'd have to go through it themselves to understand"*, and I agreed with him because it was true. Having this horrible chemical pumped into your body was just the worst thing ever. It not only affected my hair but by this time all my finger nails had indents in them through the Chemo and I suffered bad with thrush in my mouth through all the tablets I was taking and I could even smell the chemicals in my urine when I peed, it was just horrendous and I feel for anyone who has got to go through this.

Lots of people told me how brave I was going through what I went through, but I don't think I was brave, I think children who go through it are the brave ones because they don't fully understand what's going on, but they always seem to be smiling no matter how poorly they are.

"Well that's another Chemo over", I thought as I left the hospital and it felt good knowing I was half way through my Chemo.

But my happiness soon turned to tears as the weekend arrived and my husband went out to get drunk and left me on my own yet again.

I remember sitting crying my eyes out again as I felt so alone and then Todd my Son walked into the room and hugged me. He then said, *"Do you want to watch the Fox and The Hound with me?"* I just burst into tears but not in a sad way, I was just so emotional at that time that anything made me cry. But what Todd had said had really choked me up because we both love Disney films, but the Fox and the Hound was kind of special between Todd and me. I'd bought the video for Todd when he was very young and the reason being was because the fox in the story was also called Tod, but spelt with only one D.

We sat and watched that film together that day and I've never forgot what Todd did trying to make me feel happy again, he was my rock and I love him even more for that. When my husband arrived home, he went straight upstairs so I just kept out of his way. I had started to feel quite ill by then as the Chemotherapy I'd had was starting to kick in and I wasn't feeling well enough for him to start on me, so it was for the best I stayed downstairs and left him alone.

After a while I heard my husband come downstairs and go into the kitchen and I heard the oven door open and shut so I guessed he was cooking himself something to eat. Todd was out at that time as he'd gone to see his friend who only lived a few minutes away and I was pleased about that as I thought if my husband did start arguing with me at least Todd wasn't there to see it.

My husband sat in the hallway on the computer but once his food was ready he brought it into the living room to eat, but we still hadn't spoken to each other.

As he sat eating breaded chicken Todd arrived home and as he walked into the room he could smell the food, he then said to my husband, *"that smells nice what are you eating?"* My husband looked at him with a piece of chicken in one hand and a serviette in the other and replied by saying *"A tissue"* rather sarcastically.

My Son rushed out of the room as my husband had upset him so I went after him and my Son was in tears, after all he'd asked my husband a perfectly normal question. I then said, *"I've just about had enough of this"* to my husband and he replied by saying *"So have I"*. He then walked out of the living room and into the kitchen and threw his chicken all over the floor and then he left it there and went upstairs. I knew I couldn't leave it there for him to clear up the next day, I had to clear it up myself because it was chicken and I had a dog and if he'd eaten a chicken bone he might have choked. I was feeling ill and yet I was on my hands and knees picking up chicken bones and I just burst into tears. After I'd washed the floor I then phoned my sister who was in Ramsgate Kent and I told her what my husband had done, she was furious and without me knowing when I got off the phone after speaking with her she then phoned my husband's mobile and had a row with him. But my husband told her that he hadn't thrown the chicken everywhere he'd just missed the bin, just so that he didn't look the bad guy.

My husband came downstairs and said that my Sister had had words with him and then he apologized for what he'd done, but I told him that he needed to apologize to Todd as he'd really upset him, but he wouldn't apologize to my Son. I then said, *how would you have felt if your Dad had treated your Mum like this when she was ill? Throwing dinner everywhere whilst she had to pick it up"*, and he said, *"Leave my Mother out of this she's dead but you're not"*, so I replied by saying *"Well I'm sorry I've disappointed you"*.

He then left the room and went upstairs but by this time I knew then that if I got well and it was a big if, because at that time I didn't know whether I would live or die, but if I did get well I vowed to myself that when I was strong enough I'd leave him. I felt like I was coping with my cancer on my own, because he was no use to me and this was when I needed him the most.

Just before I was due to have my fourth course of Chemotherapy I asked my husband if he would take me down to Kent so that I could pick my Mother up and bring her back to Cambridgeshire with me for a few weeks. I told him I needed her with me because the doctor had said that once they put me on the new course of Chemo it would make me feel even more ill, but I knew I could probably cope on my own as I had done so far, but I was worried that my husband would start arguing with me, but I knew if my Mother was there my husband would be on his best behaviour. I was fed up with him starting on me every time I was on my ill time and I was dreading this new Chemo because I didn't know how ill it would make me feel.

My husband agreed to take me down to Kent and I spent the day at my Sister's seeing all my family and friends and then we brought my Mother back to Cambridgeshire with us.

My Father in-law took me to hospital with my Mother the day before my Chemo was due, so I could have my blood test and it was then that I showed the nurse my toe nail, it looked weird and discoloured and she told me I had an infection in my toe nail due to having Chemo and I was put on anti-biotics.

The next day I had my new course of Chemotherapy which I was dreading, but I was surprised because I didn't feel as ill as I had with the Artemis Trial Chemotherapy, but I was ill longer but not as severe if that makes any sense.

With the first three course of Chemotherapy I was ill for about three days and I could hardly do anything in that time, I just wanted to lay down, but with this new Chemo I was ill longer about five days, but I could still do work at home I didn't need to lie down all the time. I was out of breath though and I had to stop every so often when I walked anywhere.

The next day after I'd had my new Chemo my husband and I took my Mother to Cambridge, I wanted to show her how nice it was.

My husband parked his car and we walked the short distance to the Grafton Centre, but once I was there I started to feel ill and I had to sit down and a brief time later I told my Mum that I needed to go and get something to eat to stop me feeling sick, so we left the Graton Centre and went to a restaurant and had a meal. I felt awful because my Mother hadn't even had chance to look around

Cambridge, but I felt so ill, but she said she didn't mind she just wanted me to be ok.

Whilst my Mother was in Cambridgeshire staying with me she had her birthday, so I cooked a buffet and invited my Father in-law to join us that evening and although I was ill I made her birthday as special as I could.

I also showed her around the village that I lived in, but sometimes she would walk down to the shops on her own as I felt to weak. I also took my Mother to Ely and showed her the town and the Cathedral that was there.

One day whilst my Mother was still staying at my house´ my Son reminded me that he was due to go and see the pop group N-Dubz in Cambridge, I'd had the tickets for quite a few months but with everything that was going on I'd completely forgot about them. I had bought two tickets as I was going to go with Todd to watch the group, but as I was ill I decided to let his friend go with him instead. I travelled by bus with my Mother, Todd and his friend and it took about an hour to get there. Once I knew they were safely inside the Corn Exchange theatre in Cambridge, my Mother and I went and had a coffee and we waited for my husband to meet us after work and then we had a meal together. About 10pm we picked my Son and his friend up from the Corn Exchange and they'd had a wonderful time and I was so pleased because Todd had been through so much recently seeing me ill all the time.

Whilst my Mother stayed with me in Cambridgeshire my husband behaved in a respectable manner and it felt nice not having him argue with me over nothing.

But this is the side of my husband that people only saw, they never saw the horrible side of him that I saw, only my Son Todd was a witness to it all.

CHAPTER FIVE

As I sat on my own one day I suddenly remembered the survey that the hospital had given me a month or so before, so I took it out of the envelope and started to read through it. There were lots of questions regarding how I was coping with cancer and if I had all the support I needed. I decided to fill the survey out and I was totally honest about how I was feeling and how my husband was treating me so badly all through my illness.

I knew the hospital would probably question me about this but at that time I didn't care, I wasn't going to lie anymore and say that everything was fine because it wasn't.

I was doing well with my treatment and the hospital were pleased with the way the Chemotherapy was working and this gave me a boost. But I still had everything going on at home and one day I confided in the nurse at the hospital about what was happening. She couldn't believe it as every time she'd seen my husband with me he always came across as nice, but that's where he fooled everyone, he was nice to his friends or his family that lived away, but none of them saw the other side of him that I saw.

I sobbed talking to the nurse one day and she was so concerned that she spoke with my consultant at Addenbrooke's hospital, but there was nothing they could do only talk to me about everything. Even I couldn't do anything about my situation, I couldn't leave as I had nowhere to go and I couldn't just give up my house as I had my Son to think of and I was also still having treatment at hospital and I found Addenbrooke's to be a good hospital so I didn't want to change from there.

When my husband came home from work every day he was fine with me and we seemed to get on, it was only when he had an alcoholic drink that he'd change. The thing is once he started drinking at the weekend he just didn't know when to stop. I'm not against anyone drinking as I enjoy a drink myself, it's the change in personality that I didn't like because it was upsetting being shouted at all the time for no reason.

When I went to the Breast Unit the next time I saw the lady that I'd got to know over the months, the one who also had breast cancer like me. She started telling me that she had to miss her last Chemo as she'd had a toe nail infection, so then I told her I'd had an infection in one of my toe nails as well. I'm guessing hers was quite serious though being as they couldn't administer her Chemotherapy because of it. I'd have hated having to miss my Chemo, as I liked to keep up with all my treatment and tablets, I didn't want anything going wrong as the treatment seemed to be working ok by then.

One day I was asked if I would be a volunteer to have photographs taken of my breasts, it was all for research so I didn't refuse. But I remember joking with the lady photographer at the hospital, I said, *"please don't keep my face on the photograph as I don't want to be known as the owner of these boobs"*,

The lady laughed and told me that they only take a photo of my breasts, my face would not appear on the photograph.

I'd been to Addenbrooke's so many times by now that I knew my way around most of the hospital and it seemed that where ever I went I knew someone there. Whether it was a patient, doctor or nurse, I always saw someone there that I knew and it was beginning to feel like my second home.

One day as I was waiting to see a doctor in Oncology when I saw a lady who worked at a shop in the village where I lived, she was at a counter buying a drink. I walked over to her and said hello and she was really surprised to see me there. She then asked why I was there so I took my hat off to show her my bald head and I told her that I had breast cancer. She then sat down with me and told me she had been diagnosed with leukaemia. I couldn't believe it because she looked so healthy. I then asked her how she found out she'd got leukaemia and what were the symptoms and she told me that she found a lump in her groin, so she went to the doctors and they sent her to have a blood test and then she was told the awful news. She was also having Chemotherapy but unlike myself she had to have Chemo for the rest of her life. Her Chemo wasn't as strong as mine and she said she didn't feel ill with it and she didn't lose her hair either. But if I had had the choice I would have chosen to have my illness rather than hers, because at least once I'd finished Chemotherapy that was it, I wouldn't have liked having it for the rest of my life.

I got talking to a lady in Oncology who looked quite ill when I spoke to her and she asked me what kind of cancer I had, so I told her I had breast cancer. She then told me I'd be fine and she seemed quite certain of that, even though at that time I wasn't so sure. She also said she had lung and liver cancer and that it was incurable, they were just keeping her comfortable. I felt awful for her and I didn't know what to say, I just put my hand in hers and held her hand for a while. I don't know how I didn't cry in front of her that day, because I really wanted too. When I left the hospital that day I couldn't stop thinking about that lady and seeing her looking so brave had really got to me.

It made me think of how the nurses coped with all the deaths that they saw, because they must have got quite attached to some of their patients.

But it wasn't only ordinary people like me who got cancer that year of 2009, there seemed to be a spate of celebrities getting ill with it as well.

Jade Goody had passed away in March 2009, followed by Farrah Fawcett and then Sally Dynevor who plays Sally in Coronation Street also got diagnosed with breast cancer that year and then the following year Bernie Nolan, Martina Navratilova and Jennifer Saunders were all also told they had breast cancer too.

It was beginning to feel quite scary as I'd never heard of so many people with the disease.

I had asked the doctors at the hospital if my cancer was hereditary, as both my Great Grandmothers and one of my Nan's had all died from breast cancer. My Mother had always been fine but I needed to know if it was hereditary as I had a Sister who was a bit older than me and a niece who was only twenty- one at the time. But I was told it wasn't hereditary so that was a relief.

My Father in-law took me for my fifth course of Chemotherapy, it was just before Christmas at that time and the weather had started to get quite cold. I hardly left the house once the weather change, as my immune system was very low by then and to catch even a common cold could have been fatal for me.

All I kept thinking whilst I was sitting there having Chemotherapy pumped into me, was that after this one I only had to have one more course of Chemo and that was such a good feeling to have.

My Father in-law came back to my house with me that day and we sat and chatted for quite a few hours. I loved his company as he would always make me laugh and I think he enjoyed my company too.

Once he'd left to go home I sat waiting for my Son Todd to come home from school and not long after my husband returned home from work. But when my husband came home he didn't look happy, so I asked him what was wrong and he told me he'd lost his job.

My husband hadn't been at his new job very long and he was finding it quite hard trying to get used to doing something new, after all he'd only been used to his first job and he'd been there since leaving school about thirty-four years, but he'd been made redundant from that job. So, when he had to start something new he found it hard to settle in and his boss had noticed that he was struggling, so he let him go.

I was a bit like that as I liked retail work but I didn't like all the latest cash registers that most shops now had, I used to struggle with trying to learn how to use them.

I had done quite a bit of retail work in my life including retail management of a greengrocers, but everything was changing in retail and things were starting to get a little more complicated, well that's how I felt anyway.

I still had my job at the Environment Agency as a cleaning supervisor, but at that time I was still off sick.

As we sat talking over dinner I sensed my husband was relieved in a way that he didn't have to go back to that job and I was beginning to think maybe it was for the best as it's horrible being in a job that you hate, so maybe it was a good thing that his boss had let him go.

My husband still had a bit of savings so he had a bit of time to look for other work, so at least now he might find a job he liked.

As the next day arrived it was the weekend again and as you already know it was a time I always dreaded. I went shopping with my husband that day but I wrapped up warm with extra clothing on and I had a hat, scarf and gloves on that day, I certainly had no intention of getting ill.

That afternoon my husband did his usual thing of going to the pub, so I didn't say anything as there was no point. I sat with my Son and we watched video's together, that was a special time for me as being with my Son took my mind off my cancer. We'd sit and munch sweets and have our very own indoor picnic and it was nice.

But then my husband would come home drunk and spoil the wonderful day that I'd had.

When my husband arrived home that day my Son Todd was upstairs playing on his game console and I was sitting watching television. As I heard the door open I just wanted to hide away as I just didn't want to argue with him. But my husband went straight upstairs and I never heard anything from him, he must have been quite drunk though because he went straight to bed.

I sat downstairs for a few hours but as it got late I made my way upstairs to bed.

When I entered the bedroom the smell of alcohol just hit me, so I walked towards the bed and stood looking at my husband who was fast asleep and I thought how selfish he was. I then noticed he hadn't taken his sleeping pill that night as it was still on the side unit, so as not to wake him I carefully climbed into bed and it didn't take me long to fall asleep as I was shattered.

But a few hours later I was woken up as I heard my husband go downstairs. I didn't follow him I just fell back to sleep, but a while later my husband came back to bed and woke me up yet again. I still didn't say anything to him I just turned over and fell asleep again. But about an hour later I heard my husband get up and go out of the bedroom, but a minute or so later he came back in the room and started shouting at me.

He's accused me of leaving a landing light on, but I knew I hadn't left it on. I told him he must have done it but he wouldn't listen, so I said, *"If you weren't drunk you'd have remembered that you got up a while ago and went downstairs and then you came back upstairs a while later"*.

But he still wouldn't listen to me he just kept ranting and raging. It was ridiculous arguing over a light being left on and as I felt unwell I really couldn't be bothered to argue with him. I was tired and ill through the Chemo, all I wanted to do was sleep, but he wasn't going to let me do that, he just kept shouting so I ended up getting up and going downstairs to sleep on the sofa.

But a while later he came downstairs ranting and raging again and by this time I'd just about had enough. I then thought quickly and went upstairs and grabbed some of his clothes and I brought them back downstairs with me, I then opened the front door and threw them outside. I knew he'd go outside and get them and when he did I shut the door behind him and locked him out. It was the only way I could get any peace and any sleep. But it didn't end there as he stood outside banging on the door for about twenty minutes, but I ignored him. A brief time later he drove off in his car even though he was still under the influence of alcohol, but then again that had never stopped him before, as he'd already had his driving licence taken away through drink driving, but that was before we'd met.

Finally, I had some peace and I could go to sleep as that was all I wanted.

The next day my Father in-law phoned me to say my husband was at his house, so I explained to him what had happened the previous night and he wasn't happy and he said he would have words with his Son. I told my Father in-law that if he didn't stop drinking then I didn't want him back anymore and he agreed with me that this couldn't go on any longer.

A few days later my husband knocked at the door and asked if he could speak to me, so I agreed to hear him out and he promised he wouldn't drink anymore. But I didn't care that he had a drink now and again, I just didn't want him going over the top with it and then starting an argument with me. We both agreed that he'd drink in moderation and not go mad, so I gave him the benefit of my doubt.

As Christmas arrived the following week I cooked a lovely Christmas dinner and invited my Father in-law over.

We exchanged presents but one of the presents that my husband bought me supposedly as a joke was a huge box of condoms, I laughed because I didn't want to make a big deal out of it, but I was thinking how inconsiderate he was. I had been told by a doctor that once I started Chemotherapy, if I had sex I had to use a condom and that's why my husband got them. But I thought it was a strange gift because he never came near me and even though I now had condoms he still didn't bother. Don't really understand why he bought them but I just let it go and didn't comment.

We had a lovely day though and there was no arguing from my husband, but I did get tired quickly as I'd cooked all the dinner myself and washed all the dishes.

My Father in-law stayed with us until about 4pm on Boxing Day and I know he enjoyed himself because I had him laughing over the Christmas and even my husband had made it nice for him.
On the day after Boxing day I had a small parcel delivered for me and when I opened it, it was a photograph of my eldest Son and I took the year before at my Nephews wedding, my Son's girlfriend had sent it to me. When I saw it I just burst into tears, it made me emotional because he wasn't there with me, but it was a lovely thought and I did think how nice it was.
As I laid on the sofa that afternoon watching a film with my husband and my Son Todd, there was a knock at the door. Todd got up and answered it and then called to me as it was for me, but I never had anyone knock for me so I just assumed it was someone selling something, so I told Todd I was too tired to come to the door. I then heard the door close and Todd came back into the room, followed by my eldest Son and his girlfriend. I was on the sofa which had the back of it facing my Son and to this day I don't know how I did it, but I somehow got the energy from somewhere and I just jumped over the back of the sofa and grabbed hold of my Son and hugged him. Whilst I was hugging him I was crying and I looked at his girlfriend and whispered thank you to her. If it hadn't have been through her I wouldn't have seen my Son, as she drove him from Kent to see me, my Son didn't drive until the following year.
My Son Adam and his girlfriend stayed with me for a few days and then they had to travel back to Kent, but at least I'd seen them and I felt happy.
As the next few weeks passed and we were now in 2010 things seemed better between my husband and I, but I still

couldn't forget about the terrible way he'd treated me throughout my illness and I still vowed to leave him once I was well enough, but at that time I was just tolerating him but the feelings I'd once had for him had gone.

It was my birthday on the 8th January and I was due for my last Chemo that day, but because it was my birthday I'd asked if I could possibly bring it a day forward and the hospital agreed. It was snowing that day and my husband had a job interview so he couldn't take me to hospital and my Father in-law had to see his doctor that day, so I had no choice but to get the bus. Todd's school was also closed because of the weather, so he came to the hospital with me. Once I was on the bus it took about an hour or more to get to Cambridge and then I had to wait for another bus to then take me to Addenbrooke's hospital, in all it took about two hours to get there.

As I sat having Chemotherapy Todd sat beside me and we could see it snowing from the windows. I remember saying to Todd "*I hope we don't get snowed in*" and we both laughed. But the snow eased up and we managed to get home ok.

Apart from when my Mother was with me for my fourth Chemo and with this last Chemo, it was the only two Chemo's that my husband hadn't behaved badly towards me, I'd had four out of six Chemo's where my husband had been horrible to me, but I wasn't going to forgive and forget as I knew my time would come.

As the weather got worse and it had started to get quite windy a fence out the back fell, so instead of just letting my dog out on his own we now had to take him out on a lead. The fence could quite easily have been mended, but my husband didn't bother and I was too ill to even try and do it. I could do a lot of things before I was ill like decorate my whole house by myself, but the more Chemotherapy I had the weaker I became.

My husband had started drinking more now and because he didn't have work he didn't just drink at weekends, he was now drinking in the week as well.

I was dreading every time he came home and I remember phoning my Mother and asking if we picked her up would she stay here with us for a week the next month, which was February, only I was due to have an operation on my breast to remove the tumour or where it had been. But I needed someone who would help me, not someone who would just give me grief. My Mother agreed to come to Cambridgeshire and she also said she'd help my husband mend the fence, so that my dog could go out on his own without having to be put on a lead.

I explained to my husband that we had to pick my Mother up from Kent in a few weeks and he was fine about it, he probably only agreed so that he didn't have to stay at home with me whilst I recovered.

A few days before we picked my Mother up my husband went out and got drunk and when he came home he cooked himself something to eat and came and sat in the living room with me. But a brief time later he started trying to push for an argument, he told me that when my Mother comes up he wasn't going to mend the fence with her, so I just said ok don't worry, but he kept saying it just so I would snap back, but I didn't and I think that must have annoyed him more, but I just couldn't be bothered, I knew what I had planned once I was well and that kept me going.

I travelled to Ramsgate Kent with my husband so I could then see the rest of my family and we brought my Mother back with me and then the day arrived for me to have my operation.

My husband drove my Mother and I to Addenbrooke's and we had to be there about 7am so we all had to be up early that morning. After I had booked myself in we were told to take a seat in the waiting room and then I had to have a blood test done and I was explained to in more detail what would be happening to me that day. I was taken to a ward and given a bed and I sat talking for hours to my husband and my Mother and then I had to be taken to another part of the hospital for a scan. My Mother offered to come with me, but I don't think she was expecting to see what the nurse did to me and neither was I. I had an ultra sound scan and the tumour could no longer be seen, as it had shrunk so much, but the clip was still in place so they knew where the tumour had been. As I lay on the bed the nurse told me she had to put a metal rod into me, so that the doctors knew where to operate and she then gave me an injection to numb my breast, but it didn't work that well as I felt everything. I just lay there having this long piece of rod pushed into my breast and I could see by the look on my Mother's face that she looked concerned. Once again, I didn't make a sound I just let the nurse do her job, but it did hurt and I did have tears running down my face. Once the rod was in place they had to leave part of it hanging out of me, but they tapped it up so that I didn't catch myself on it and then I was taken back to the ward. My Mother then told me how brave I was, but like I said before I didn't really think I was, I thought the brave ones were children or people that had been told that they were terminal, they're the brave ones.

A few more hours went by and then two doctors came to my bedside to speak with me and one of those doctors was the guy that had first diagnosed me with cancer, he was a lovely man and he was to be my surgeon that day.

He examined me and then draw a cross onto my breast just to make sure they operated on the correct breast, but seeing as I had a metal rod sticking out of me that should have been conclusive enough.

I wasn't scared that day because I knew they were going to take the cancer completely out of me and I knew this was the beginning of my road to recovery.

An hour or so later I had a pre-med and then I was taken down to theatre and I remember how friendly the staff were, they were amazing and they tried their best to put my mind at ease.

Once I'd had the operation I was put into a recovery room for a while, but when I got back to the ward my Mother said I'd been down there quite a few hours. But to me the time had gone quick, I'd been put out under anaesthetic and the next thing I knew it was all over with.

A nurse there kept coming to my bedside and taking my blood pressure and temperature and I remember I suddenly wanted to be sick, so they quickly grabbed a cardboard type bowl, but once I'd been sick I just kept on going and the nurse got quite concerned about me. I'd had quite a high dosage of Morphine pumped into me and it was that, that was making me sick. The nurse gave me some sick tablets to calm my sickness down a bit, but it didn't stop me.

A few hours went by and then the surgeon came to my bedside to speak with me. He told me he'd removed the area where the tumour had been and part of the new area just to make sure he'd got it all and he said he couldn't find any more cancer in my breast. I was quite emotional by then and I remember shaking his hand and I looked him

straight in his eyes and thanked him, after all he'd saved my life.
I was still being sick and the nurse told me that if I was sick again they'd have to keep me in overnight, but somehow, I stopped being sick so they let me go home. But I'd only been in the car a few minutes when suddenly I wanted to be sick again, so my husband had to stop the car and I got out and was sick in the curb of the road.
When I got home I just laid on the sofa with a duvet over me and I was very tired by then. My Mother was also tired as she'd been up early and I also think the worry of me tired had her out even more.
After they'd eaten an hour or so later my Mother decided to go up to bed, but she asked my husband if he could take the dog out before he went to bed and he agreed. But when my husband told me he was going to bed I said have you taken the dog out and he said no I'm not going out there as it's raining hard and he went upstairs to bed. So I had to get up and take the dog out myself and stand in the rain with my dressing gown on, even though I'd just got out of hospital after having an operation.
I slept on the sofa that night as I was worried in case my husband turned over in the night and knocked my breast, but I slept well and felt a lot better the next day.
When my Mother got up I told her that my husband didn't take the dog out the night before and she was angry, but I told her not to say anything as it would make things difficult for me once she'd gone back home, so she kept quiet but she did say to me you need to leave him and come back to Ramsgate and I agreed with her, but I couldn't do anything yet as I still had radio therapy to have in about two months' time. On the day my Mother went home I decided to spend a week in Ramsgate as it was the

school half term, so Todd and I stayed at my Sister's house and we had a really nice time. I met up with Adam my eldest Son and I visited a few friends that I hadn't seen for a while.

I even had to see a nurse at the surgery where my Sister went, because a few days after having my operation I was told I needed to have the dressing changed, but the nurse there was lovely and she was very gentle as she cleaned the wound and she even showed me my scar before redressing it. The surgeon had done a neat cut and it wasn't much wider than a hair, just a little bit wider but it wasn't as bad as I thought it might be, so I was quite pleased with that.

Whilst I was in Kent Todd met up with some of his old friends and when he came back to my Sisters he started to get upset. He said he didn't want to go back to Cambridgeshire, as all his friends and family were here in Ramsgate, but we had no choice but to go back and I felt quite bad for him having to go back to a place he hated and to a step Father who was constantly rude to him, calling him names all the time. But Todd would have never of stayed in Ramsgate without me and he knew I had to go back to finish the last of my treatment.

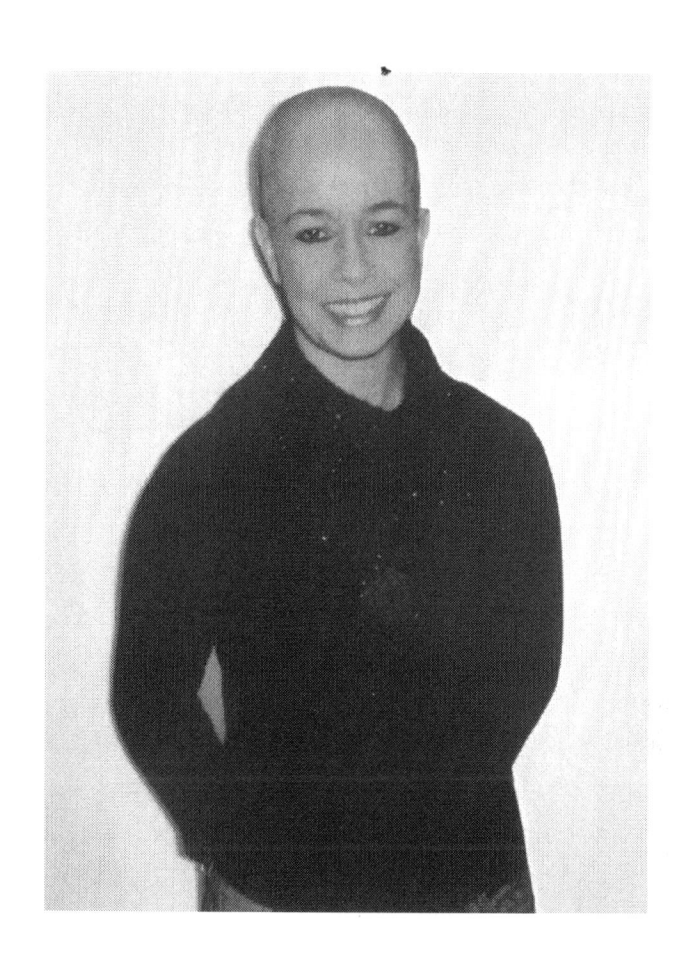

CHAPTER SIX

When I arrived back in Cambridgeshire I phoned my Father in-law to see if he wanted to come over to our house for dinner the next day and he was pleased to except.
I hadn't seen him for a while so I was looking forward to him coming to see us the next day and I cooked a lovely Sunday roast.
I still had a few hospital appointments the following week but nothing to serious. I was given some tablets called Tamoxifen and I had to take one tablet every day, but that was fine by me as that was nothing compared to all the tablets I had to take whilst on Chemo. I was told I had to take one tablet a day for the next five years, but after three years they would change my tablets to a different one.
I had to wait for two months before starting my radio therapy, but in that time my Father in-law would often come and visit me and as my husband was no longer working we could get to see my Father in-law more often as well.
I remember one day my Father in-law mentioned about the gold charm bracelet that he'd given to me on the day I was diagnosed with cancer and he asked why he hadn't seen me wearing it. But I told him that I would wear it but only on special occasions, as I didn't want to damage it, but it was safe upstairs in a tin with my other jewellery. I never thought anything more about it until about a month later and I went upstairs to have a look at it, but when I opened the tin the charm bracelet had gone. I knew instantly that my husband had taken it, as he'd already complained that it belonged to him and that his Father had no right giving it to me. I searched everywhere for it and I eventually found

it in a tin which belonged to my husband, he had other jewellery in there as well which had also belonged to his late Mother. I then took the bracelet out of the tin and hid it, after all his Father had given it to me, but I never mentioned to my husband that I'd taken it back, I thought he can find out for himself later.

My hair had now started to grow back, I had just a little bit coming through, but it was a start. I still wore hats though but things were finally getting back to normal for me and I started to feel a lot happier in myself.

I still had some hospital appointments but nowhere near many as I'd had before.

I had to have a MRI scan quite a few times and I also had a scan to check the density of my bones, because Chemotherapy can affect people's bones, but I was told I had the bone density of a thirty-year-old which pleased me.

Once April 2010 arrived I had to start having Radio Therapy, I had to have it every day for three weeks but not at weekends.

As I lay on the bed I was told I had to have the machine lined up accurately and rather than mark my body with pen every day, they told me they had to tattoo three small dots on my body. I had one either side of the top half of my body and one in- between my breasts, it looked like I had a small blackhead on my chest, but it was so tiny it didn't really notice that much.

I then went through a small tunnel in the machine, very similar to an MRI scan and I could see a small red light, I guessed that was the laser type of light. The machine then started and I could hear the nurses explaining to me what would happen, even though they were now in a separate room as they couldn't be with me because of the radiation.

I didn't feel anything I just closed my eyes and relaxed and it took about twenty minutes for the Radio Therapy to work.
The Radio Therapy was nothing like Chemotherapy as it didn't make me ill, I just felt tired about ten minutes after I'd come off the machine, it felt like I'd had a sleeping pill, but I could cope with that.
It was a bit of a drain having to travel forty-five minutes every day to hospital and then back again, but what could I do? It had to be done.
My husband wasn't so bad to me now that I was getting stronger, maybe because he knew I didn't have to put up with him anymore, but I still needed him because I had hospital every day.
Once I had finished all my treatment my friend Kim came up from Kent to see me, we'd known each other since school when we were eleven years old.
We walked down the village together and I showed her around and we also sat down outside a pub and had a cold drink down by the river.
It was nice having her there as I didn't have any friend's much where I lived, although my next-door neighbour would sometimes pop in for a quick chat, but as I said before she didn't live in that house, they'd bought it to do it up and let it out, so I didn't see her very often.
I took my friend Kim to Ely one day and we sat down by the river there as well, but it was better than in my village as they had lots of boats and ducks around. The ducks were quite friendly and would often walk up close to people and it was lovely to watch them.
When we were walking back towards the town we suddenly saw a Mother duck with about six ducklings following behind, but they had to cross the busiest road in

Ely to get back to the river. I panicked as they crossed into the road and I ran into the middle off the road and stopped the traffic and I did the same on the other side of the road until they were safely back on the path again. My friend laughed at me but I couldn't stand and watch them be run over.

Whilst my friend was staying with me Todd had his birthday and my husband also had his the following day, so I did a buffet on both days and invited my Father in-law over on my husband's birthday, so he could be there too. It turned out to be lovely on both days and my husband was like a different person whilst my friend was there.

I confided in my friend about the way my husband had behaved towards me whilst I'd been ill and I also told her that he never came near me sexually, so she said let's go shopping and she advised me to buy a sexy outfit to wear in the bedroom. I didn't feel sexy at that time because I had very short hair, only a slight bit showing through, but my friend told me not to worry, she said I looked beautiful. That night I put on the sexy outfit and showed my husband, he said it looked nice but he was sorry he was tired. I then walked out of the room and took the outfit off and threw it in the bin, I never tried to get him to make love to me after that as I didn't see the point. All I wanted was to be made to feel like a woman again, but he couldn't even do that for me, I was so upset.

One day whilst I was down the other side of the village my friend noticed that the pub had a sign-up advertising that they were having a foam party the next day, so she said she would like to go. I wasn't sure because I hadn't been out for ages and I still didn't feel like the old me with my hair so short, but she wasn't going to stop going on about it until I agreed to go.

Todd stayed at his friend's house that night and my husband, Kim and I went to the pub and I've got to admit I had a lovely time. My husband introduced me to some of the people in the pub as he already knew them, as he was quite a regular down there by this time and they all made me feel welcome.
I remember one lady who was nice, she was Scottish and her name was Heather, she spoke to me quite a bit.
When my friend eventually went home I was quite sad because I felt alone again and it had been nice having someone to confide in. But all my treatment was now over so as far as I was concerned things could only get better.
I went back to work after my friend had gone back home, but I found it hard to keep up with everything I needed to do there and in the end, I had to give the job up. I think I went back to work to soon as I'd not long finished my Radio Therapy, so I was still not fully recovered from my treatment. I decided to take some time out and find a job once I felt strong enough and this break gave me time to get over all what I'd gone through those past eight months.
My Father in-law had given me some money for Christmas and my birthday for me to learn how to drive and I'd saved it for when I finished all my treatment. I then booked up to have driving lessons with a guy who lived in the village. But after about six lessons I started hating it, I was a nervous driver and I should have really taken lessons in an automatic, but my husband advised me otherwise. But eventually I gave up driving because I was getting to stressed and I was worried I'd make myself ill.
A few days after I gave up driving my next-door neighbours asked my husband and I if where'd like to go out with them to the pub one evening, so we agreed and that night the lady asked me how my driving was going, so

I told her I'd given it up and before I could say anything else my husband said, *"yeah she's useless"* but my neighbours husband said, *"no she isn't"* and stuck up for me.

I tried to ignore my husband's comment and just act like everything was fine, but he'd upset me yet again and to do that in front of people had devastated me, but when I told him about it the next day he said he couldn't remember saying it, so I just left it at that.

As the weather got warmer on my Son's school holidays I spent more and more time in Ramsgate as I needed to see my family and my eldest Son Adam. One night my Sister and her husband and her eldest Son had planned a night out, my eldest Son was also going to be there and they asked me to come along. I couldn't drink a lot maybe one or two drinks because I still had to build myself up to be strong again. But as I got in the pub my Son ordered him and his friends some drinks in small shot like glasses and my Son offered me one. I said no because they look like shots and he said they weren't they were just a liquor, so I believed him and had one, but my Son began to laugh as he'd given me a shot of Sambuca. Within a few minutes, I couldn't even see in front of me clearly as the shot just hit me, I could have throttled my Son because it ruined my night and my Sister and her husband had to take me home. My Son hadn't meant to ruin my night he just wanted me to have an enjoyable time, but I didn't need a shot to enjoy myself, just hearing music I liked was enjoyment enough for me. I do like a drink but I didn't want to drink so soon after my treatment had finished, I needed to get over all what I'd been through, after all in eight months I'd had two operations, Chemotherapy and Radio Therapy.

On our first wedding anniversary, my husband booked us into a chalet at a pub for the evening. I happened to come across this beautiful pub one day on the internet and it looked amazing, I never would have dreamt my husband would book it for me. We looked around the village for a while and in the evening, we had a meal at the pub. I had a chicken salad and it had a vinaigrette dressing on it and it tasted lovely, but after about twenty minutes after eating it I suddenly felt ill and I thought I was going to collapse. I told my husband I needed to go back to the chalet which was situated outside next door to the pub, so he said, *"ok but I'm going to stay here"*. So I walked back to the chalet on my own and got into bed and it was only about 7.30pm by then so it was still quite early. I must have slept well though because I only woke up when my husband came back and by then it was gone midnight. I soon fell back to sleep but the next morning I was covered in a rash, it looked a bit like German Measles. We left the chalet and I asked my husband to take me to hospital as I needed to find out why I had a rash and the doctor told me I had an allergic reaction to something I'd eaten and he gave me some antihistamine tablets. But I didn't feel ill then I felt fine I just had a rash and needed to get it cleared up. A few days later the rash had gone and I don't really know what had caused it, but whatever it was it had ruined my night away for my anniversary.

I was starting to walk about a bit more now and I wasn't so out of breath as I had been, but I was fed up with just being in the village or going to Ely to get my shopping, I wanted to do more now that I was stronger. I asked my husband if he would come swimming with my Son and I, but he refused as he said he didn't like swimming, but I'd seen a video of him when he was abroad once and he was in a swimming pool then. So I suggested about going to the cinema, but again he said he didn't like going, so by then I guessed that he didn't want to go anywhere with me, or do anything apart from go to the pub, but I didn't think it was fair on my Son not being taken anywhere and I was limited where I could go because I didn't drive. I then told my husband that I was going to tell his Father that he had refused to go anywhere with us and he soon changed his tune, he then said choose somewhere then but not swimming or the cinema, so I told him I wanted to go to Colchester Zoo. I'd been there a few times before as I once lived in Colchester for six years and I loved it there. My husband agreed to take me but I had to pay for the petrol and entrance fee, but I didn't argue as it was my idea.

I had a wonderful time at the Zoo that day and so did my Son. I had even fed a giraffe and an elephant, it was lovely feeding them and the elephant sucked the food up with his trunk and it felt just like it was being sucked up by a hoover, but a bit slimier. Once I'd fed the elephant I said I've got to do that again, so I queued up again to feed it and that was the highlight of my day.

We saw tigers and lions that day and one of the tigers was white, it was beautiful. They also had Zedonks at the Zoo, they were half Zebra and half Donkey, they had grey bodies and stripes on their legs.

I had such an enjoyable day that day I'd even forgotten that I'd been ill, the thought hadn't even crossed my mind that day, it was brilliant.

After that day I made my husband start taking us out a bit more, it didn't hurt him after all he spent enough time in the pub when he wanted.

One day I went to Huntstanton in Norfolk with my husband and Todd. It was a seaside town and it had a few amusements there and rides for everyone. Todd went on a few rides but he wanted me to go on the Waltzer with him as he knew that was my favourite ride, so I agreed and it was great fun, but after I got off I had to sit down as I felt quite sick, I'd never felt ill on the waltzer before but I guess my body couldn't cope with everything so soon after my treatment.

We then went and bought some fish and chips and they were lovely and we had a look around the town there. They had quite a few nice little shops there which sold gifts and I bought Todd a poster of Al Pacino and I bought my eldest Son Adam a dummy made from candy, but it was blue and said Everton on it, which was his favourite football team.

In the Aug of that year Todd's friend was going to Haven holiday park in Norfolk and as I had got to know his Mother she asked if I wanted to come with them. It didn't cost anything as she'd already paid for the caravan, so I spoke with my husband and he said go. All I needed was money for food and any spending money. We went for five days and Todd and I had a lovely time, I think this was what we needed to have a break away. My husband had promised to take me on holiday once my treatment had finished, but that never happened.

Whilst we were there we played mini golf but I wasn't very good, but I did like playing ten pin bowling and air hockey.

We had a Chinese takeaway one night and we took it back to the caravan, it was lovely because we'd bought a variety of Chinese food, so we had quite a choice of what to have. Todd even had a go at fencing whilst we were there and I was pleased that he was out enjoying himself for a change.

Most evenings we would watch people sing and watch comedians perform, it was very entertaining.

As we drove back home we passed Bernard Mathews house and it was beautiful a lovely place surrounded by countryside.

When we finally arrived home, I was a bit sad because it was back to reality once more, but I had had a lovely time and I know Todd had too.

As it was the summer holidays I also took Todd to Ramsgate again and Todd was out most of the time with his friends from Kent. But even though I didn't see much of Todd throughout the day, it was nice that he was out enjoying himself. He'd spend days down the beach or in the park, but it was better to have him like that than being stuck indoors on his game console.

Although I'd stay at my Sister's house when I went to Ramsgate, I still used to pop up to see my friends who lived at the top of the road near where I used to live and I'd also meet up with friends from school.

Once the summer was over I then had to spend lots of money on a new school uniform for my Son and my savings were going down fast as my husband didn't contribute anything towards my Sons upbringing, maybe because he wasn't his Father he didn't think it was his place.

We had my husband's friend come to our house one Sunday, so my husband decided to have a barbeque so we all went shopping to get some food. But I needed a few things for myself, but as we got to the checkout my husband's friend noticed that he only paid for his food and he pulled me up about it, he asked why my husband hadn't paid for my food as well, so I said I don't know he's always done it like this. His friend said *"Ahh bless you"* and offered to pay for the few bits I had, but I said no its fine. I think he was quite surprised because we were a married couple, we weren't living as lodgers in a house share, but that's how it felt sometimes.

I was beginning to think I was more like a Mother to him than anything else, after all I did all the washing, cooking, cleaning etc, but we had no sex as a married couple, it was like a marriage of convenience, but it wasn't what I'd moved from Kent for. I wanted more than this in my life and since being ill I knew there was a life out there for me, but only I could change things and that was to move back home where I belonged in Kent.

I told my husband I wanted to move back to Kent and he said he wouldn't come with me if I did, so I told him I didn't care as I didn't want to be with him anymore and then things turned nasty as he started shouting at me.

I'd already confided in his Father about moving back to Kent and although his Father didn't want me to go, he told me he didn't blame me at all.

But a few weeks later my husband told me that he'd been InTouch with my housing association and unless he agreed I couldn't move. I was devastated as the house was still in my name only and my husband had savings from the sale of his flat so he could quite easily find somewhere else to live, but no he just wanted to make things difficult for me. I just had to get on with it and put up with things the way they were and I started to get quite depressed.

As Christmas was almost upon us again I decided to go to Kent with Todd and stay at my Sister's, after all I hadn't had a Christmas with my family for quite a few years and I also wanted to spend a Christmas with my eldest Son Adam. I didn't care that I wouldn't be there with my husband and why should I have considered him anyway, he hadn't considered my feelings in the past.

I was now getting stronger in my body but also in my ways and I knew I didn't have to put up with everything like I had done when I was ill. I could suddenly do what I wanted just like he had and there was nothing my husband could do about it.

I had a lovely time that Christmas and all my family were together, my two Sons, My Mother, Sister, brother in-law, brother and Sister in-law and I even got to see my nieces and nephews as well whilst I was there and I was happy. When I returned to Cambridgeshire my Father in-law told me that was the worst Christmas he'd ever had and I felt bad for him because I hadn't made it special for him and he'd been so good to me over the months, but I needed to see my family too and I wasn't trying to be unkind to him, I would never have done anything to upset him.

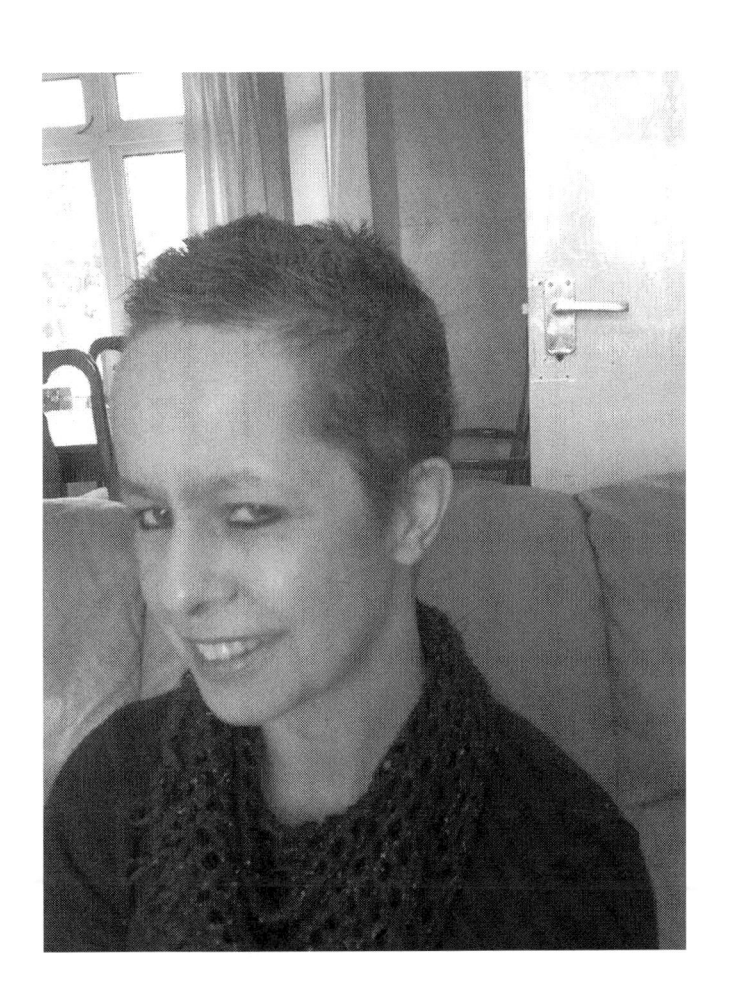

CHAPTER SEVEN

It was now 2011 and the weather was freezing but I used to speak to my Father in-law most days on the phone to make sure he was ok and so did my husband.
One weekend my Father in-law came over for dinner and after we sat and chatted for quite a few hours and everything was fine. But a few days later when my husband and I tried phoning him there was no answer, so we both assumed he'd gone out to the shop or maybe he had a doctor's appointment. So we left it a while and tried phoning him again later, but there was still no answer. So we were getting a bit worried by now and we both decided we needed to go to his house which was about a thirty minute drive, just to make sure he was ok.
When we arrived my husband who had a key to his Father's house, tried to open the door, but the door was locked from the inside. So now we were really concerned and we started banging on the windows, but still no one came to the door. My Father in-law was eighty-eight by this time so we knew anything could go wrong with him at that age. We then asked some neighbours if they'd seen him but no one had, so we had no option but to call the police. We didn't dare smash a window and break in just in case he was lying dead inside the house, we didn't want to be accused of foul play or anything like that, so we left it to the professionals. When the police arrived, they tried banging on the door but there was still no answer, so they then phoned Addenbrooke's hospital to see if he had been admitted without telling anyone, but he hadn't so we knew he must be inside the house. As we all went around the back of the house once more, suddenly my Father in-law

came to the door. But he didn't look well at all. The police then left and my husband and I went inside the house and it was then that my Father in-law said he felt poorly, but he didn't know what was wrong with him. My husband contacted his doctor and my Father in-law was admitted into hospital and after quite a few tests it was confirmed that he had pneumonia.

My Father in-law wasn't happy that he had to stay in hospital as he was very independent, but we told him he was in the best place and that they would soon have him well again. He was put on anti-biotics but he wasn't the easiest of patients, sometimes even refusing to take his medication, but we managed to persuade him that it was in his best interest to take his medicine and he listened to us. My husband and I seemed to put all our differences aside at that time and we went to the hospital together every day. My Father in-law went off his food but I told him unless he started to eat more he wouldn't be allowed home and I used to spoon feed him just to make him eat and he used to laugh thinking it was funny, he was such a stubborn man but he was lovely.

My Father in-law was in hospital about two weeks, then one day we had a phone call to tell us we could now come and collect him as he was being discharged from hospital, so we made our way to Addenbrooke's about 7pm that evening. When we arrived at the hospital my Father in-law was sitting in a wheel chair with his bag ready to be taken home, so my husband spoke to the nurse, but whilst he was talking with her I sensed something was wrong with my Father in-law. He just didn't look right to me and I asked him if he was ok, but he told me he felt very ill. So once my husband came back over towards me I then explained to him that his Father wasn't well enough to come home.

My husband again spoke to the nurse but she seemed to think he was fine, so we had no choice but to take him home. Once we were at my Father in-laws house I told my husband that I didn't think his Father should be on his own as he looked quite ill and I said if you don't stay with him then I will, but he agreed to stay with his Father, so my husband took me home and then drove back to be with his Father. But that night my Father in-law took a turn for the worst and started bringing up bile, so my husband called an ambulance and my Father in-law was rushed back to hospital. I knew he didn't look right when we picked him up from hospital, but the nurse was adamant that he was fine.

My husband stayed at the hospital for most of the night, then he came home the next morning to get some sleep as he hadn't slept all night.

The hospital did tests the next day and it turned out that my Father in-law had a hernia and they asked for us to come to the hospital as they wanted to operate on him that night. When we arrived I sat beside my Father in-law whilst my husband spoke to the nurse and it was then that my Father in-law told me that he was worried about having the operation because of his age, so I said I'll speak to a doctor about his concern. A while later I did explain to the doctor that he was worried about having the operation in case he didn't pull through because of his age and the doctor said he would get the surgeon to phone us. Whilst my husband went to get a drink an hour or so later, the telephone on the side rang, so I had to answer it and I spoke with the surgeon and he seemed to think despite my Father in-laws age he needed to have this operation and that his heart was strong enough to take it. So I then told my Father in-law that I'd spoken to the surgeon and that he had nothing to worry about and he cupped his hand on my face and said you're so good I do love you and he smiled with a relieved look upon his face. When my husband came back I explained to him what the surgeon had said to me, but instead of being pleased for his Father, he was annoyed because I'd spoken to the surgeon and he hadn't. But I wasn't going to get into an argument at the hospital, so I just said well it's been done and he's going to be fine and I left it at that.

We stayed with my Father in-law until he was taken down to surgery and the doctor told us as it was late we should go home and phone in the morning to see how he was, but obviously if anything went wrong they'd contact us immediately, so my husband and I made our way home.

We didn't hear anything from the hospital that night so we had guessed that the operation had gone well, but my husband and I were up early as we wanted to phone the hospital to see how my Father in-law was.

My husband spoke to a nurse and she told him that the operation was a bit more complicated than first thought, the hernia had attached itself onto his bowel so it was quite a difficult operation.

Thinking about it now I don't know how the nurses didn't see that my Father in-law was still poorly when they sent him home, because I knew straight away something wasn't right and I'm no doctor.

Later that afternoon we made our way to the hospital and when we got there my Father in-law was lying in bed bringing up bile and the smell was awful, it smelt the whole ward out, but I tried to help him by rubbing his back and wiping his mouth. But he just couldn't stop bringing up the bile and I had to ask the nurse for more sick bowls as he kept filling them up. My husband walked over the other side of the ward and stood looking out of the window because he couldn't stand the smell and even a nurse turned her nose up as she walked past, but that annoyed me because if she couldn't cope with the smell she shouldn't be in that job. I was the one helping him and yes, the smell was awful, but he needed help and no one else was bothering. It was horrible for him being in a ward with other people and the nurses hadn't even pulled the screen around him, so everyone could see him bringing up bile. It was quite undignified I thought, so I pulled the screen around his bed to give him some privacy. But It got so bad that I ended up calling a nurse over and asked her to give my Father in-law something to stop him bringing up the bile and eventually he was given something to help him. I don't know how long he'd been like that before we arrived, but I wasn't happy as the nurses didn't do anything to help him until I intervened.

A brief time later things calmed down and my Father in-law stopped bringing up bile, but he wasn't looking at all well and he kept saying things that hadn't really happened, it was as if his mind had gone slightly, but I put it down to the medication that he was on.

I sat holding his hand and kept telling him he was going to be fine, but he looked quite poorly and to be honest I wasn't sure myself that he was going to get over this operation. Once my Father in-law stopped bringing up bile my husband came back towards us and sat the other side of his Father, but all my Father in-law wanted was to go home. We kept telling him he couldn't go home just yet as he wasn't strong enough, but I don't think he appreciated us saying that.

Before we left to go home I gathered up my Father in-law's clothes to take them home to wash and then I hugged and kissed him and we left the hospital.

All the way home I couldn't stop thinking about how ill he was and for the nurses to sit there and do nothing was appalling.

My husband phoned my Father In-laws Sister that evening to let her know what was happening with her brother, only she lived away so unless we explained to her what was going on she'd be none the wiser.

The next day when we arrived at the hospital my Father in-law was standing beside his bed arguing with a doctor, but then he saw my husband and I and he told us that they were trying to kill him. I calmed him down and he got back into bed, but it was then that my husband and I realized that my Father in-law was not in his right mind and we spoke to the doctor about it. We were told because of his age some operations can affect patient's minds, the doctor told us he sees this kind of thing all the time. But it wasn't nice for us watching my Father in-law shouting and making up things that wasn't true, but in his mind, it was.

There were quite a few other patients in the ward and a few of them spoke to us, but they were not too seriously ill and one man was due to go home later that day.

The next day when we visited the hospital we were told that my Father in-law had now been moved to another ward and when we found where it was we saw that he now had a room of his own. Not long after we got there a lady brought the patients lunch around to them, but my Father in-law hardly touched his food, so I once again spoon fed him and made him eat a bit more.

Whilst we were there he pointed to a young nurse and told us she had eighteen lovers and ten children, but we knew this wasn't true, it was just his mind playing tricks on him again, but it did make us laugh.

After my Father in-law had been in hospital about a week we were taken into a room by a consultant and he told us that my Father in-law was very poorly and he wanted to know if anything happened to him would my husband want him resuscitated. It came as quite a shock as we thought he was on the mend, but obviously not. My husband didn't know what to say but only he could make that decision.

We went to the hospital every day and my Father in-law had been in hospital for a few weeks by now, but although he recognized my husband and I, he still came out with things that hadn't really happened. One day he told us that his car had blown up so now he couldn't drive it, but we knew it was safe at his house in the garage.

I took some old photographs to the hospital one day to see if he could identify the people in the pictures and he was telling me that one was his wife and another his Sister, but I think eventually he got fed up because when I showed him another photograph he told me it was Andy Pandy and burst into laughter. We all laughed but I guess his mind had come back that day, but he still hadn't lost his sense of humour.

My Father in-law had his eighty- ninth birthday in hospital and we didn't really know what to buy him, as there wasn't a lot you could get someone who was in hospital. I suggested we buy him a new jumper because he liked looking smart, so we bought him two new jumpers and I also got him a balloon with birthday boy written on it and we sang happy birthday to him when we got to the hospital.

A few days later his Sister came to visit him and I think that perked him up.

After being in hospital for a few more weeks my husband was told that we needed to find his Father a care home to move into as they had done all they could for him at the hospital, but he wasn't well enough to return home. I didn't like the thought of him going into a home but we couldn't have him live with us because we had no downstairs bathroom facilities and I wasn't strong enough to look after him as I couldn't have lifted him up to wash him.

My husband decided that we had no choice but to get him the care that he needed and he looked around for a nice care home for his Father.

I didn't even think about leaving my husband at that time, as my thoughts were only on my Father in-law. I thought a lot of him and he had been good to me when I was ill the year before, so now it was my turn to be there for him.

A few weeks later my husband found a nice care home for his Father and we looked around it and everyone seemed friendly there, but my Father in-law hated it and he told me he didn't want to be there, I felt awful but there was nothing I could do.

My husband didn't visit his Father everyday like he had when he was in hospital and I couldn't get there by myself as I wouldn't have known how to get there, it was about fifty-minute drive away and I didn't know the area.

My husband started to spend more and more time at the pub and his drinking once again became a problem, but I wasn't ill anymore so when he started on me I could now give as good as I got.

I remember one day he came home drunk and he brought up about the charm bracelet that his Father had given me.

He told me he knew I'd taken it from his tin and he wanted it back, so I said your Father gave that to me and you were the one who took it from me and you had no right, I just took back what was mine. But he wouldn't let it drop so in the end I said, *"if you don't stop I'm going to phone your Aunt and tell her exactly how you treated me when I was ill and even now you're still doing it"*.

I then picked up his mobile phone and made out I was going to phone her if he didn't stop arguing, but he suddenly pushed me against the wall and put his hand around my throat, but I still didn't let go of the phone. He then let go of me so I gave him his mobile, but I told him that when I see his Father next, I'm going to tell him how badly he is behaving towards me because he doesn't want me to have his late Mother's bracelet. But my husband said, *"leave my Father out of this"*.

Of course he didn't want me telling his Father everything because he knows his Father would be annoyed with him. The next day I told him I think he should move out as he could now go and live at his Father's house, but he was adamant that he wasn't going anywhere. We didn't speak after that but he left the house to go and visit his Father, but he never even asked me if I wanted to go with him. I stayed in all day and when my husband returned he told me he'd spoken with his Father and his Father didn't want to see me anymore. I didn't believe him because his Father thought the world of me, he was just saying that so I couldn't visit his Father anymore and tell him the truth. We had a big row and I told him to leave and I meant it at that time. He put a few items of clothing into a bag and then he suddenly went into my out-house and made a phone call, I stood listening and it was then I heard him talking to his cousin and he told her I'd stolen his Mother's bracelet, I couldn't believe what I was hearing, I was livid and when he got off the phone I told him I'd heard everything and I said, *"you'd do anything to make yourself look the good guy"*. But I knew the truth and so did his Father.

He then left and stayed at his Father's house and I didn't hear anything from him, but I was really upset that I couldn't go and see my Father in-law. That was one of the most hurtful things my husband had ever done to me and he'd done a lot of hurtful thing over the years, but to stop me seeing his Father was not only cruel to me but also to his Father.

I hadn't seen my husband for a few weeks but then I got a telephone call from him asking if he could come and collect some more clothes, so I agreed as I would never stop him taking anything that belonged to him. When he arrived, he spoke to me in a civil manner and I did him, but I still wasn't happy about not seeing his Father and I told him so. He then said get ready and I'll take you over there now, so I didn't hesitate, I quickly changed my clothes and we made our way to the care home. But when I got there the lady who run the home hugged my husband, but didn't even acknowledge me, so I guessed my husband had obviously said some awful thing about me to her, but I didn't know what and I never said anything whilst I was there.

When I walked into the room where all the patients were seated, I saw my Father in-law sitting in a chair and when he saw me he smiled, I then bent down and hugged him and he burst into tears. He then said, "I've missed you so much, I do love you".

I looked at my husband as I was furious and I said, *as if your Dad didn't want to see me, just look at him and see how upset he is.*

My husband didn't answer me but he knew what he'd done and the lies he'd told.

I sat holding my Father in-laws hand and spoke to him and he was happy to see me. But when it was time to leave I didn't like leaving him, it was awful as he watched us walk away and I felt terrible.

When we got outside I had an argument with my husband for not letting me see my Father in-law and I also wanted to know why the lady at the care home was hostile towards me, but he made out he didn't know, but I could see right through his lies and when I got home I told him to take his clothes that he needed and leave.

About three days later I was woken up by the telephone ringing, but when I answered it, it was the funeral director wanting to know if they could take my Father in-laws body from the care home, or does my husband want it to stay there a while longer. I was shocked and I explained to the lady that my husband was at his Father's house, so she said she'd call him on his mobile. I couldn't believe my Father in-law had passed away and yet I'd only seen him three days before and I couldn't believe my husband hadn't even told me so I phoned him. As he spoke to me he cried and I felt quite sad for him, so I told him to come back home and I'd help him sort everything out, so he did.

We both went to the care home and saw my Father in-law and then we had to go and pick up the death certificate. It stated that he had died from a urine infection and I remember him telling me it hurt when he peed.

Over the next few days we registered the death and arranged the funeral with the funeral directors. He was to be buried with his late wife not far from where they used to live.

Before my Father in-law was buried I bought him a St Christopher and I placed it in his hand, I thought as a St Christopher is the patron Saint of travellers, this would make him safe on his journey.

I told my husband I'd do all the food and I spent hours the day before cooking everything and making sure it was a nice send off for him. All we had to do was take the food to his Father's house the next day, as that was where the wake was being held.

My husband phoned his cousin that evening and I overheard him saying that I was the dutiful daughter in law but not the dutiful wife. I couldn't believe he could say something like that after all what I'd done. Not just because I'd cooked the food and helped him arrange the funeral, but I was there for my Father in-law when he was ill, wiping his mouth when he was bringing up bile and washing his clothes when he had had an accident. Yet all my husband did was run me down. When he came off the phone I told him I had heard what he'd said and he just laughed, so I said, *"how can I face your family knowing you've slated me to them and told them I stole your Mother's bracelet"*, but he didn't answer me. I then told him that he could take the food to his Father's house the next day, but I wouldn't be attending the funeral.

I then sat in my living room and slept downstairs that night and the next morning my husband got up and started loading up the car with the food that I'd cooked. Then he came back into the house and told me he was leaving to go to his Father's house, I just looked at him and cried and I told him I'd never forgive him for this, but he just turned and walked out of the house.

Todd my Son sat and hugged me but I just couldn't stop crying.

Then as I sat thinking about all what my husband had done to me, but how caring his Father had been and I thought why shouldn't I be at the funeral.

I told Todd to get ready and I got changed and I then ordered a taxi to take me to my Father in-laws house and when I got there I told my husband I didn't have any money on me so he had to pay the £28 taxi fare. He didn't argue he just paid it, but I knew he wouldn't argue in front of his friends and family anyway.

Everyone there were nice to me but there were a few people that were a bit offish towards me, but I knew in my mind that I hadn't done anything wrong and if my husband had said otherwise then that was up to him. I just carried on laying out the food and I held my head up high and my Father in-law had a lovely send off.

My husband's Aunt stayed late helping me clear up and wash-up the dishes and she was lovely to me, but she didn't know anything about what I'd gone through with my husband in the past and I never told her, only my Father in-law new the whole truth but he was no longer here to back my story up.

My husband asked if he could stay at my house that evening and I agreed after all I didn't think it fair for him to be on his own after he'd just buried his Father.

CHAPTER EIGHT

As the next few months passed things seemed to be a little bit better between my husband and I, but I was still adamant that I was going to move back to Kent. I couldn't forgive him for the way he'd treated me and to lie to his family about me stealing his late Mother's bracelet was just unforgiveable.

My Father in-law had left me £2000 in his will and he also left me his car which was one of the old vintage mini's, but it was in excellent condition and it was also automatic which I preferred. I don't think my husband was happy about me getting the car, but that was his Father's wish and this time he couldn't accuse me of stealing it.

Because I couldn't drive I left the car in my Father in-laws garage, as I knew it would be safe in there and my husband didn't mind me leaving it there, probably because he thought I'd never be able to take it.

One day in September 2011 I had Todd's friend at my house, so I asked my husband if I paid the petrol would he take us out to the seaside for the day, I thought it would be nice just to get out and go somewhere different for a change.

My husband agreed so we took the boys to Hunstanton and they had a wonderful time going on all the rides. They also had Candyfloss and fish and chips for lunch and it was an enjoyable day. We spent a few hours walking around and it was such a pleasant change to be by the seaside.

As it started to get chilly we decided to make our way home. We dropped Todd's friend home in Ely and then we all went back to our house, but my husband then decided to go to the pub, but I stayed home with Todd.

A few hours later as I sat quietly watching the Wizard of Oz my husband came home drunk. He went straight upstairs and into the bedroom and a few minutes later my TV switched over. My husband had switched it over from upstairs, but when he did that it switched the downstairs TV over. I called to him to let him know I was watching the Wizard of Oz and I wanted to see the end of it, so I switched the TV back again. My husband then came downstairs and started to unplug the Sky box, so I asked him what he was doing. He told me that he was taking it upstairs so that he could watch it and I couldn't. I said don't be silly and tried to take it off him, but he then told me I was psycho. I just saw red by this time and said if you think I'm Psycho I'll show you Psycho and then I grabbed the Sky box and broke it up, I then told him if I can't watch TV then neither could he. He stormed out of the room in temper and went back upstairs.

A while later I had a knock at the door, it was the police. My husband had phoned them to try and get me arrested for criminal damage, but when I explained to the police what he had done and that the house was in my name they took him away, so it had totally backfired on him this time. But now that the police had been involved it had done me a favour, because if I had any more trouble I only had to call them, as I knew they would stop him coming to my address.

The next day I phoned my housing association to see how I stood if I wanted to move back to Kent and they said now that my husband had been left his Father's house, he could live there and I didn't need his permission to move.

I then started looking for exchanges on the housing sites, but there wasn't many available wanting my area, so I just had to keep looking.

I had now started buying new things for when I moved and I had bought a brand-new table and chairs which I'd put in my outhouse, it was still boxed up but ready to move as and when I found a place.

One day I had a knock at the door it was my husband and a police officer, my husband had come for his belongings, so I let him in and he took what he could manage, but the larger items such as his wardrobe, bed and sofas had to be put onto a lorry later.

I helped my husband pack his belongings and I knew there was no going back this time, but I was relieved it was like a weight had been lifted from my shoulders and I felt happy. I think I should have got him out months before, but there was always an obstacle that stopped me.

A few days later my husband came back to take his larger items and he had a guy with a lorry to help him, so I just let them get on with it and I stayed out of the way. But later that day after my husband had taken all his belongings he phoned me and told me he'd also taken part of my brand-new table that was boxed up and I couldn't have it back until I gave him his late Mother's charm bracelet. I couldn't believe he'd stooped that low, but I just wanted rid of him so I told him he could have the bracelet, as I wasn't prepared to keep arguing over it. The next day he brought part of my table back and I gave him the bracelet, I didn't speak to him I just gave it to him and closed the door.

My Son Todd and I were fine we had each other without any hassle and it was nice.

A few weeks later I received a letter from a solicitor on behalf of my husband. In the letter, I was asked to sign an agreement so that I couldn't claim anything from my husband's saving from the sale of his flat. I didn't want anything from my husband but I thought I'd make him sweat a bit, after all he'd put me through hell over the years. I wrote a letter back telling his solicitor that I had no intentions of signing any agreement and I felt great sending it off.

About a week later I received another letter from my husband's solicitor telling me that if I didn't sign the agreement, they'd have no option but to start divorce proceedings. I think my husband had forgotten that I was well by this time and I didn't have to take everything he dished out at me anymore. I then made an appointment with a different solicitor and I started divorce proceedings against him.

Once he realized what I'd done he phoned me and cried begging me not to take any of his savings, but I just told him I didn't want anything from him, all I wanted was for him to sign the divorce papers once it was finalized and he agreed. I felt for once in all the time I had been with my husband that I was finally in control and I didn't have to take his nonsense anymore.

As the next few months passed Christmas was almost upon us once more.

I had been living on my own now for just over three months and yes, I did get lonely at times, but it was better than having arguments constantly.

I was still looking for a move and I did have a married couple from Ramsgate come and look at my house, but they pulled out not long after which was disappointing.

I was dreading Christmas this year as I knew I couldn't go to my family because I had my dog to consider and I couldn't take him with me as my Sister had her own dog and I doubt very much if they'd have got on. But I had to make the most of it for Todd's sake and I tried my hardest to make it special for him.

I remember cooking a small buffet for me and Todd on Christmas Eve and we had planned to play a quiz game. We had both written question on pieces of paper for each other to answer, but if we got a question wrong we had to do a forfeit. It was quite funny and we had a good laugh. I remember one of the questions I'd written for Todd to answer, it said, "*Who was the original presenter of the Generation Game?*", and of course the answer was Bruce Forsyth, but Todd said it was Fruce Borsyth. We both realized at the same time he'd got the name muddled up and we couldn't stop laughing. But because Todd got it wrong he had to do a forfeit and I made him sing a song with his tongue hanging out and it was almost impossible but we cried laughing.

I bought Todd lots of nice presents and we had a lovely Christmas dinner on Christmas Day and we watched films together in the afternoon.

My eldest Son Adam phoned me on Christmas Day and again on Boxing Day, he told me he was going shopping on Boxing Day as he didn't have to work and he sounded pleased because he could go to the sales.

As I sat with Todd later that day my Son Adam phoned me again and I asked him if he had bought anything nice in the sales, but he said no I didn't bother going in the end, so I asked him why. He then told me to look out of the window and when I did he was sitting outside in his car. I was still on my mobile to him at that time and I just looked out and said, "*Oh my god, Oh my god, Oh my god*",

I was so excited and pleased to see him and he just made my Christmas that little bit more special. Even now Todd often mentions about that Christmas and just because it was only Todd and I together Christmas Eve and Christmas Day, it didn't stop us having fun, it was lovely. As the New Year arrived it was now 2012 and I was still no nearer to moving, but I was getting quite depressed by this time as all I wanted was to be back in Kent and be near my family and friends, after all I had nothing to keep me in Cambridgeshire and I was beginning to feel like a recluse.

I was still quite out of breath but I put it down to the cancer tablets I was on, I knew it couldn't be the Chemotherapy anymore as I'd finished my treatment. But I just carried on as normal and just got on with it.

I used to chat with my friends quite regularly on social media, that was the only thing that kept me sane, otherwise I'd have gone crazy because the only person I was seeing was Todd.

I was looking for work but I just couldn't get a job and the lady at the job centre was nice and I used to often chat with her about my circumstances and she knew how desperate I was to move back where I belonged.

One day whilst I was on social media I saw an advertisement advertising a Thanet Council Housing group, so I applied to join and then I could see if anyone was looking to live in my area.

I was on the list for a transfer which meant I could be moved from one council to another, without having any other tenants involved, but it went by a point system and I had no chance. Even after all what I'd been through and needing to be back with my family I was told I'd have to wait at least two years on their list. Therefore I tried other ways to see if I could get an exchange with someone else, because I wasn't prepared to wait two years to move or even longer.

I looked every day on that site but still I didn't have any luck. Then one day I saw a lady on the site who I was friends with on social media, she used to live opposite me in Ramsgate when I lived there. She had since moved to Margate and she had a three-bedroomed town house, but she wanted to move to Sussex, so I emailed her to see if she was interested in doing a three-way swap, that way someone from Sussex would have my house, I would have my friends and my friend could then move to Sussex. It sounds complicated but it was the best solution I could come up with, after all I didn't have any other options. My friend Gail was pleased that I was interested as she was in the same boat as me, finding it impossible to get a mutual exchange, but all we needed now was to find someone who was interested in moving from Sussex to Cambridgeshire.

A few weeks later Gail emailed me telling me she might have found someone who wanted to move from Sussex to Cambridgeshire, so she contacted the lady and was waiting on her reply. It took a while but the lady did eventually reply and she seemed very keen to move, so all we had to do now was view each other's houses. The lady from Sussex came to view my house first and she seemed very keen and then I went to Kent for the day and viewed the house in Margate. It was a lovely house set on three floors and it was nicely decorated throughout, it even had a small room that was bigger than some single bedrooms and it had a radiator in it and a window, so really it was a four-bedroomed house, but the housing association only classed it as a three. It also had three double bedrooms as well, which not even private houses get, as usually houses with three bedrooms have two doubles and one single bedroom.

It was lovely and it was only a five-minute walk to Margate High Street and about a ten-minute walk to Margate hospital and bus routes were a few minutes' walk away, so everything was on hand. The garden wasn't very big just a back yard, but it was big enough for my dog or for anyone to sit in. I didn't mind the size because I didn't like gardening much anyway.

I told my friend Gail I was very interested so all we needed now was for her to go to Sussex to view the other lady's house.

The following week Gail went to Sussex and she was also very interested in the lady's house, so now we had to get the ball rolling and fill out the exchange forms.

It was quite a lengthy process and we had a few hiccups on the way, but it took about two months in all to finalize the move.

I was so excited about moving and as I'd since spoken to my husband on the phone I told him about the move. We seemed to get on ok being apart and that suited me. He even offered to drive me down to Margate on the day I move and as I didn't drive I knew I'd have to find someone from Kent to come and get me, so I excepted my husband's offer.

I was still going ahead with the divorce as nothing had changed in that sense, but it was nice that my husband and I were now being civil to each other, but I still couldn't forgive him for the way he'd treated me whilst I was ill, but I didn't bring it up to him again as it wasn't worth the hassle.

The worst part of moving was the packing and having my house look a mess, but I knew I was doing the right thing and I knew I'd be so much happier.

As the lorry arrived it was only small and I told the driver I didn't think he would get all my belongings onto it, but he reckoned it would be fine so I let him and the removal guys get on with it. But a few hours later I was told I would have to leave all my garden tools behind and my barbeque, as there was no more room on the lorry. I wasn't very impressed as I'd already given him an infantry of what items I had, so really, he should have brought a bigger lorry, but it was too late now so I had to leave some items behind.

As I sat in the car and we started on our journey back to Kent I was so relieved to be leaving Cambridgeshire. I had no happy memories there, as all I'd seemed to have was bad luck and bad health, so it wasn't hard for me to say goodbye.

I did have one lady who I was sad to leave, her name was Dorothy and she lived a few doors away from me in Cambridgeshire. She'd often knock on my door to see if I was ok when I was ill and she was the one who bought me a thermometer so that I could check my temperature regularly. I still receive a letter from her now and again and I always reply.

As we travelled in the car I phoned my friend Gail whose house I was moving into, I just wanted to make sure everything was ok with her, but she was panicking as she'd broken down half way to Sussex. What a nightmare for her and she had little ones in the car as well. But she managed to get someone to pick her up and take her the rest of the way to Sussex, so everything worked out well in the end. Gail had given me a front door key but she'd also left the backdoor unlocked for me just to make things easier, but I had to go in through the back entrance anyway as it was the easiest place to park.

Adam my eldest Son phoned me a few times whilst I was travelling down to Kent, he was at work but he still wanted to know how far away I was, as he wanted to know I was safe. When I arrived at my new home my Son Adam was there with his friend, he hadn't got work after all, but he didn't tell me as he wanted to surprise me. He'd been sitting outside for ages waiting for me, but I laughed and told him you could have gone in because the back door is open.

He looked at me and said, "*You're joking*", but he saw the funny side of it in the end.

Once the lorry had been unloaded my husband left to go back to Cambridgeshire, I was a bit sad because of the way things had worked out between us, but I had no regrets. This was a new beginning for me and I was going to make the most of it, I'd been stuck in a village that I hated for four years and suddenly I felt free and it was a great feeling.

My friend Tracy came around who I knew from school since I was five, she helped me sort a lot of my boxes out, whilst Adam helped set my TV and DVD up. As I looked around my house I was so happy, there wasn't anything that I didn't like about it and Todd was also thrilled especially as he had the biggest bedroom in the house, it was huge I'd never seen a bedroom that big before.

Adam didn't say much because he wasn't one to show his feelings very much, but I know he was glad to have me back home again and his brother Todd.

Over the next few days I had so many visitors wanting to see me and my new house and it was so nice to have company again, I'd missed not having people around me and it had got quite lonely for me.

I was quite busy the next few days as I had to get Todd into a secondary school and I also still had forms to sign with my housing association and I also had to book in with the job centre as I needed some money. I still had a bit of savings but I knew it wouldn't last long, as I still needed things for my new home. I had to purchase three double beds for each bedroom and I put Todd's single bed in the small room, the one that they didn't class as a bedroom. I also needed new wardrobes for myself as I'd given mine to Todd, but I wanted to decorate the whole house before I bought anything. The house wasn't in a horrible state as Gail had left it decorated lovely, but I wanted to put my own stamp on it, so that it felt like my home and not someone else's. I decorated Todd's bedroom first in yellow and slate, as he wanted a New York style bedroom and when it was finished it looked amazing. I'd put posters of New York and gangsters on his wall, he had a New York rug, lampshade and bedding set and black curtains and everything went well together and he was really pleased with the result.

I decorated my bedroom next and then the small room, I worked my way from top to bottom, but I left the hallway and landing until last, as I had a long hallway and two sets of stairs so I knew that would be the hardest job of all.

As I decorated I was still quite out of breath and I started to get tired quite quickly, but I put it down to over working as I didn't stop all day. I even had to book in a dentist and a doctor as I needed my cancer tablets prescribed every two months, so I had lots of things going on at that time. But as the weeks went by I felt like I had flu but without a cold and I slept most of the day, well three out of seven days I slept and on the days I didn't sleep, I was decorating my house. I wanted it done because I knew once I got a job

I wouldn't have time to finish it. I also needed to update the address on my CV, but because I didn't have a printer I asked the jobcentre if they could help me. They booked me in to see a guy at the jobcentre who helped people with CV's, but once I was there he took me in a room and spoke to me for about an hour and then he told me to meet him at the library the following Wednesday as he had a CV club held there every week. I wasn't happy because I'd assumed he was going to help me with my CV that day, but he didn't he just wasted an hour of my time talking nonsense. But I still went and met him the following Wednesday and I was taken into a room with about twelve other people, but I'd noticed that there were no computers in the room, so I thought how is he going to help with my CV if there are no computers. I sat quietly waiting to see what he had to say and he brought out a piece of wood with a long nail hammered slightly into it and he told us they we were going to take it in turns to balance another nail which would be upside down on top of the nail in the wood. Then he said he was going to put us into groups and we would have to make things with straws. I was fuming I wasn't going to sit there and make things like a child at playschool, so I got up and told him I wasn't prepared to do that and I walked out. I came back home and phoned the jobcentre straight away and complained, because by then I was forty-eight years old not two years old and I told them that it was humiliating what they expected people to do and the guy at the jobcentre apologized to me. I did eventually get an updated CV but what a performance I had trying to get one.

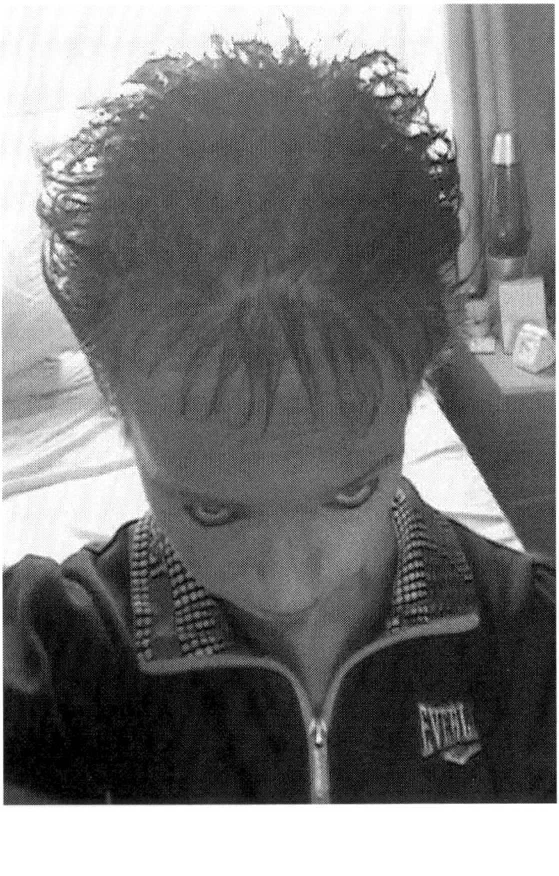

CHAPTER NINE

I'd now lived at my new house just over a month but I was still feeling exhausted all the time, so I eventually made an appointment with my doctor. I saw a lady doctor and she was nice and friendly and I explained to her how I was feeling tired all the time and out of breath, so she did the usual things like blood pressure, temperature and checked my breathing. She then told me to go home and pack a bag and go straight up to A & E and when I get there they'd be expecting me as she was going to contact them, so all I had to do was go to the A & E reception and give them my name. I then asked why I had to go to hospital and she said that I could possibly have a clot on my lung. I was shocked as I'd been all through breast cancer and I was just getting my life back on track and now this happens. I left the doctors and made my way home which wasn't far and then packed a bag and walked the ten-minute walk to the hospital. When I got there, I explained who I was and that the doctor had sent me and they told me to take a seat in the waiting room. But I was only sitting there a few minutes when a lady came and got me and took me to a ward. I was told I could either sit in bed or on the chair beside the bed, so I chose to sit in the chair and the nurse put a name band onto my arm. She then told me she'd be back soon to take some blood.
I sat in the chair thinking *"why me? Hadn't I been through enough over these last few year's"*.
As I sat there I thought I'd better let my eldest Son Adam know what was happening, so I phoned his mobile but he couldn't talk long as he was at work. I explained to him that I'd been admitted into hospital with a suspected clot on my lung and he said, *"ok don't worry I'm sure*

everything will be fine", and then he had to go. But as I was sitting reading a brief time later my Son walked into the ward. I was surprised and I said to him, "*Aren't you supposed to be at work?*". He replied by telling me that he told his boss he had to leave and he said, "*You're not going to be on your own this time whatever the outcome is*".
I was so moved by what he had just said to me and it felt good that I had people around me who cared, it wasn't going to be like before when I lived in Cambridgeshire.
A while later I had blood taken from me, but until they knew the results I wasn't going anywhere. But then I remembered that Todd was still at school and I didn't know if he had taken his key with him that day, so I phoned my Sister and I asked her if her husband and her could pick him up from school later and bring him to the hospital and I then explained to her why I was there. But she didn't hesitate she agreed to pick Todd up so that was one less worry for me.
A few hours later I had a doctor come to my bedside to speak with me and he asked what my symptoms were, so I explained to him I was breathless, feeling exhausted all the time and sleeping a lot. He then asked if I'd lost any weight and I remembered that I had lost quite a bit, but I put it down to being on the go all the time, as I always kept myself busy except for when I had to sleep.
He took notes and then he said he would come back a bit later, so I was still none the wiser what was wrong with me. I was given something to eat in the hospital and by that time I needed it as I was starving, I was eating quite a lot at that time but I was still losing weight not gaining any.
I sat talking to my Son for a few more hours and then the doctor came back and told me I had to have a scan, so I

followed him to where I had to go. It didn't take long to have the scan and I was soon back on the ward again.

As it started getting later I was beginning to get worried as I didn't want to have to stay in hospital overnight and then my Sister arrived with Todd and she stayed for a while and then left leaving Todd with me. It was nice having both my Sons with me, but I felt sorry for Todd as he'd seen me ill so much over the last few years and this didn't help. Eventually the doctor came back and he said I've got some good news and bad news, I was a bit worried by then. He then told me I hadn't got a clot on my lung, but whilst having a scan they did find a small nodule on my lung, but that wasn't causing me to be out of breath. Apparently, the nodule was so small it wasn't anything to serious to worry about, but they still needed to keep an eye on it every so often, so I would have to go back to hospital to have a scan now and again. But the reason I was out of breath and so tired all the time was because the blood test had shown that I'd got an over active thyroid, therefore my heart was racing constantly as if I was working 24/7. I then had to make an appointment with my doctor so that she could refer me to a doctor at the hospital who deals with thyroid. I was relieved that I hadn't got a clot on my lung but I knew I still had more hospital appointments to have so I wasn't pleased about that.

After I'd spoken to the doctor I was told I could go home, so Adam gave me and Todd a lift home and then I phoned my Mother to let her know my news.

I didn't stop over the next few days as I had to make a doctor's appointment and when I spoke to her she told me that I would probably have quite a lot of hospital appointments to attend, as well as coming back to see her over the next few weeks. But then I got worried because I was still looking for work and what would happen if I got a job and then had to take time off because of hospital appointments, I don't think a new employer would appreciate that. So I phoned the jobcentre and explained my situation to them and I was advised to apply for E S A. Which stands for Employment Support Allowance. It meant I could still get a bit of money but it gave me a bit of time to get well before I had to find a job, so that was good as I knew I couldn't be in two places at once and I wasn't feeling well enough to do a lot anyway.

Before I went to the hospital I received my divorce papers and when I wrote on Facebook that I was now divorced lots of people phoned me to see if I was ok, but I was fine I was happy that I was no longer married and I felt free again.

I soon managed to get an appointment at the hospital, but before seeing the doctor I had to have another blood test taken and then a few days later I saw the consultant. He then checked my eyes and made me put my hands out in front of me, he told me he was checking my hands for tremors and he also told me I not only had an over active thyroid, but I also had Graves' Disease. I didn't really know what that was but I was going to check it up on the internet when I got home. The consultant also told me that the reason I had an over active thyroid was caused through stress. It must have started when I was in Cambridgeshire because that was when I first became out of breath, it must have been caused through all the stress I'd been under with breast cancer and with the way my husband treated me. I then felt I still wasn't free from him at that time.

The consultant gave me tablets to take for my thyroid and I was also given beta blockers to slow my heart rate down and I had to go back to see him a few weeks later.

When I got home I looked up Graves' Disease and it said it's an autoimmune condition, which means the immune system mistakenly attacks the body. It attacks the thyroid and causes it to become over active and Graves' disease can eventually cause some people to have bulging eyes, so now I know why the consultant checked my eyes.

I had started to feel low again but there was nothing I could do, I just had to take the medication I was prescribed and hope for the best.

The tablets took about three months before they finally kicked in and started working, it was an awful time and I had felt so ill and tired, I thought that it was never going to go away. But I eventually picked myself up and got myself well, but I still had to take thyroid tablets for over a year, I couldn't just stop taking them because I felt a lot better, otherwise I'd have been ill again.

At that time, I was still finishing off decorating my house and because of being ill it ended up taking me about six months to finally finish decorating, but it looked lovely in every room and I was pleased with what I'd achieved.

I was still on E S A but I was trying hard to find a job as I didn't want to have to go back on Job Seekers and sign on. I was applying for anything really as all I wanted was to work now.

I finally got a call for an interview at a school, it was to do cleaning five hours a day Monday to Friday. I didn't particularly want to go back to cleaning as I'd done it before and I hated it. I've always said I think cleaners work harder than what their given credit for and I think they should be paid a lot more than they get and not just because they work hard I think they should be paid more because it's a horrible job as well.

I've done a few cleaning jobs in my time but I've also worked in retail and even done retail management, but I couldn't get a job in retail so I had to take what I could get. I had the interview and I got the job and although it wasn't my ideal job it was better than having to sign on, besides it had taken me eight months to get a job as I hadn't heard from any others that I'd applied for, so it was better than nothing.

I remember starting that job 28th January 2013 it was cold and had been snowing and I had to travel by bus from Margate to Ramsgate every day.

I had a lady called Sonia show me around and explain to me what I had to do. I was given the job of cleaning all the toilets and there were about seventy-four toilets in the school, it was the worst job ever but I just got on with it. I remember being introduced to a few ladies who were a lot younger than me, but I got on with all ages so that wasn't a problem.

I remember one day walking down a corridor with Sonia and Carlene and I said to them we ought to buy ourselves pink jackets, like the Pink Ladies from the film Grease and then we could walk along the corridor together and say *"We're gonna rule the school"*. They both laughed and then I started laughing.

I had a nice lead cleaner who was only about twenty-three, I got on well with her and we'd often work together. Even though it wasn't a very enjoyable job we all made the best of it and still had a laugh at times.

I had a lovely boss and he was very considerate when I needed time off to go to hospital appointments, because I not only had my thyroid being checked, I still had to have blood tests and I was still having breast examinations regularly as well. But he was lovely about it so sometimes if I'd finished my shift and someone on the afternoon shift had phoned in sick, I would sometimes stay on a bit later to help. I didn't mind because it helped my boss out and he was good enough to let me have time off when I needed, so I was just repaying him the favour.

I'd only been there about a month when I had to see the breast cancer nurse at the hospital and by then I'd been on Tamoxifen tablets for three years, so they had to change them to a different tablet for the next two years. It was only one a day so it didn't really bother me, but I still had to take my thyroid tablets as well at that time.

After being at the school a few months I started to get bad pains in my joints, every time I bent down I had trouble getting back up as it hurt and my fingers were hurting, but I put that down to wear and tear because I used to ring cloths out every day when cleaning the toilets and sinks. But one day I noticed my ankle was swollen but I still went to work and carried on as normal, but then I sat talking to my boss one day and he noticed that my hands and fingers were swollen and he said I should get it checked out in case I'd got arthritis, so I made an appointment with my doctor and she referred me to hospital and I had to have an X-ray on my hands. I was told I could have rheumatoid arthritis and that's what I was being checked for.

But when I came home from work one day I got thinking that surely if I had rheumatoid arthritis it wouldn't have come on that quick and it got me thinking. Then I remembered that I'd not long changed my cancer tablets from Tamoxifen to these new ones, so I looked up the side effects and everything I had with swollen joints to aching and pain in my bones come under the side effects of these new tablets. I made an appointment to see my breast cancer consultant and I explained to her what was happening, so she took me off those tablets and put me back on Tamoxifen and I have been fine ever since, but where I would have normally been on tablets for five years in all, because they've had to change them back I now must take Tamoxifen for ten years.

I told my boss and he was pleased that I'd finally sorted the problem out and I continued as normal with my work at the school.

Some of the kids in the school were nice but others were quite unruly, they'd put paper towels into the plug hole in the sinks and leave the taps running and then there was a flood which needed to be cleaned up. Other times there would put paint all over the toilet seats and graffiti on the walls and it all took a lot of time to clean and sometimes it would put me behind with my work.

Some of the kids would bring loom bands to school and they used to be everywhere on the floor and others would walk maltesers into the carpets, it was just awful and we could never actually catch the person who did it so that was annoying.

The only good thing about that job was that I got holidays off as the job was term time only, that was the best thing about working there.

I only worked Monday to Friday so it was nice to get the whole weekend off, but as Summer was almost upon us my boss asked if I'd work at the Summer fair which was being held on a Saturday. I agreed because he'd been good to me over the months, but I did tell him I didn't want the job of litter picking and he agreed I wouldn't be given that job.

When I arrived at the school some of the teachers had stools with games to play and some of the kids sold drinks, but then I saw my boss and asked him what he wanted me to do and he told me to ask the guys who I worked with. I was then given the job of litter picking and I went back over towards my boss who was sitting sun bathing and said you told me I wouldn't be doing litter picking, but he laughed and said you'll be fine. I didn't really mind and I did see the funny side, he'd conned me into working that day without telling me I'd be litter picking, but I had a plan to get my own back.

A few hours later things had quietened down at the fair and it wasn't that busy anymore, so I went into one of the cleaning cupboards and picked up an empty plastic bottle and washed it out thoroughly and filled it up with water. I then went back outside and crept up towards my boss and I squirted him with water, he jumped up and said, *"you cow"*, but I just stood there laughing.

Later that day as I was picking up the last of the litter I suddenly found a £5 note, so I then walked back over towards my boss and said to him, *"I don't mind doing the litter picking it's been quite good, especially now that I've found £5* and I stood waving the £5 note in front of him. He then called me a jammy cow and it made me laugh even more. I bet when my boss knew he was going to give me the litter picking job he had a right laugh, but I was the one laughing in the end and it turned out to be an enjoyable day.

After working at the school for about a year my boss left and I was gutted because I got on well with him and we had a new lady boss start work at the school. But when we were introduced to her she started to tell us about all the changes she was going to make and that we were no longer allowed a break time like we'd always had and she told me that if I needed to go to hospital at any time I'd have to

make the time up. If we had any queries she didn't seem to listen and she was rude all the time.
I was in the cleaning cupboard one day and my new boss came in to fill up a bucket, but she spilt water everywhere and then she looked at me and said, *"Oh well you can clear that up"*,
I was gob smacked I couldn't believe how rude she was and on another occasion, she asked me to help clean one of the canteens, so I swept the floor with a broom, but she told me I had to use a flump, that's one of those kinds of sweepers that they use in hospitals. But I'd used one before and I found it easier using a boom. I told her this and I said I can't get used to using a flump I prefer to use a broom and she told me to get used to it. One of the ladies who worked in the kitchen heard her and she spoke to me about it after, telling me how rude my boss was and I agreed. But I couldn't say anything because I didn't want to lose my job.
My boss was mostly based at Dover but we never knew when she was going to turn up in Ramsgate, but when she did everyone's mood changed for the worst. No one really liked her and many times I went to HR to complain about her. She wasn't a people person and her attitude stunk. I'd done management in the past but I was always nice to the staff, it makes people work better in a happy environment. All the girls started getting down at work including myself and it wasn't a pleasant place to work anymore, but as work was low in Thanet, we just had to get on with it.
I'd been feeling quite well by now and my thyroid tablets were working, but I was starting to worry that if I got to stressed that my thyroid might start up again. Once I finished being on my thyroid tablets the consultant told me that I shouldn't have any stress, because if I did I could

relapse and then I wouldn't be put back on tablets I'd have to have radioactive Iodine. That I didn't fancy, just the name of it sounded horrible.

I tried to just get on with my work and keep out of her way, but it wasn't always that easy.

Sonia my friend who had shown me around when I first started there had been at the school about five years and she couldn't cope with the stress anymore so she found another job, followed by my lead cleaner. It was awful as all the people I enjoyed working with were leaving, but I couldn't seem to get another job even though I was trying my hardest.

Then one day I found out that everyone's rota had changed. I had been taken off toilets and had been given an extensive list of jobs to do and they were to be done in a certain time limit, but the other ladies only had half the work I had to do. I was fuming and even the other ladies couldn't understand why I'd been given so much work, whilst they only had half as much. I ended up getting upset so I made an appointment with my doctor and when I spoke to her I burst into tears, she then signed me off work for severe depression. I was so scared that I was going to relapse with my thyroid, that I decided I would take the advice of my doctor and take some time off work.

But I needed to sort out about my rota later because I wasn't prepared to go back to work until they took some of the work load from me, it was just too much what they'd given me.

I had about a month off work and then I went to speak to HR and I showed her the paper with the list of jobs I was told to do. But she told me I didn't have to do all that work every day, she said I only had to do only some. But my boss had told me differently, she'd expected me to work miracles.

It was almost the Summer holidays so I told HR I'd come back to work after the holidays and she agreed that I needed that time to get me over my depression.

I left the school feeling happier knowing that my boss couldn't expect me to do as much work as she thought and I had HR behind me backing me all the way.

CHAPTER TEN

I was at home one day when out of the blue I got a message on social media from my cousin whom I hadn't seen for thirty-two years. He now lived and worked in Hong Kong, he worked in a bank there in Kowloon.
He said he was coming to England and could he come and see me and of course I said yes as I hadn't seen him for so long. I was a bit nervous because I didn't know anything about him anymore, or what he was like. But the day he arrived it was as though he'd never been away from me and we hit it off straight away.
He came to my house one afternoon so I showed him around Margate town and then that evening we went out for a meal with my two Sons and the rest of my family and it was a lovely evening. When we got back to my house we had a few glasses of wine and we just sat talking until quite late.
I told him about my illness and how awful things had got between my husband and I and he looked quite concerned. He then said maybe you need a holiday and he said I could stay with him and his wife in Hong Kong if I wanted. I couldn't believe he'd asked me to go out there as I'd only ever been to Paris and I'd never been on a plane before. I was a bit scared of flying by myself because I'd never flown, so I asked if my eldest Son Adam could come with me and my cousin said yes.
My cousin stayed the night at my house and he left the next morning as he had other relations and friends to meet up with, but we kept in touch by phone.
After he'd gone I looked on the internet for flights to Hong Kong and as soon as I found one that I thought was

reasonably priced I booked two tickets. We were due to fly out just over a month later and I couldn't wait.

My cousin who also had a house in the Philippines said whilst we're out in Hong Kong, he would also fly us to the Philippines for four days, from a Friday to a Monday. I was so excited as things like this never happen to me, it was like a dream come true.

Todd didn't mind not going because he didn't have a passport, but I promised to take him another time. My friend agreed to stay at my house with Todd so he wasn't alone, so now I was just counting down the days.

I went out and bought myself a lot of lose dresses as my cousin had told me it would be very hot in Hong Kong and I bought plenty of shorts and t-shirts too.

My cousin sent me photographs by text of Hong Kong and it looked amazing, he'd even send me a view from the office that he worked in and it looked fantastic, as he worked in the tallest building in Hong Kong.

The holiday couldn't come quick enough for me as it was just what I needed.

When the day arrived, I rushed around making sure everything was right before I left. I'd tidied the house, made sure there was enough food for Todd and my dog and I also left Todd some money just in case he needed it.

Adam's girlfriend picked us up and drove us to the airport, but on the way up to London I felt sick, we had to stop at services so I could use the toilet and I was quite ill by then. We then had something to eat and my stomach settled down, so we got back in the car and made our way to Heathrow Airport.

Adam's girlfriend dropped us off and then left straight away, so I then walked into the Airport and Adam showed me what I had to do, after all I'd never been to an airport before, it was all new to me.

Once we had given in our luggage we then made our way upstairs to customs and then to the waiting area, but we had quite a few hours to go before we could board our plane as we were very early.

We had a look around the shops and got something to eat and drink just to pass the time, but it seemed to take forever for the time to go. Our flight was at 10.30pm and it was a twelve-hour flight and because of the time difference between England and Hong Kong we wouldn't arrive until 5.30pm Hong Kong time the next day.

I text Todd and a few friends just to pass the time, but it went real slow, I even bought a couple of magazines to read thinking it would make the time go quicker, but it seemed like the hands on the clock weren't moving.

I was getting tired by now and yet I still had a twelve-hour flight to go, but I was still extremely excited.

Once our flight number came up and we were told which number gate to go to my heart started to race, but what I didn't realize was that I then had to sit in another waiting room before boarding the plane. *"Was I ever going to get on it"*, I thought.

But about twenty minutes later we were called to board the plane and as we got on Adam told me to sit by the window, as he'd been on a plane lots of time so he knew what to expect. As everyone boarded the plane and got comfortable, I then waited excitedly for the take off and as the plane started moving I began to laugh and I got the giggles bad, probably just nerves but I couldn't stop. I loved it when we took off and I didn't feel scared, but maybe I was without realizing.

Adam put a film on his TV to watch but I was too excited to concentrate with watching a film, so I listened to my music on my mobile and put the TV on so that I could see where the plane was and I watched as it flew through different countries.

I did try and sleep a bit on the plane but I only dozed, I hardly had any sleep that night probably because I was over excited.

We had an evening meal on the plane and then as it got morning we were given a breakfast.

As we got closer to Hong Kong I couldn't stop looking out of the window and I could now see some of the tall skyscrapers situated in Hong Kong, it looked amazing and I was overwhelmed.

As we landed all I wanted to do was get off the plane and view this beautiful country. My cousin met me at the airport and once I saw him I felt relieved because I knew I wouldn't get lost now.

As we made our way outside the heat just heat me and I looked at my cousin and smiled and I said, *"Who put the heating on?"* jokingly, and he laughed

It was about a forty-five-minute drive from the airport to my cousin's apartment, he lived in Mid-Levels which was an expensive part of Hong Kong. As we travelled in my cousin's car he pointed to different buildings and told us what they were, it was like being in another world.

My stomach had settled down a bit since the day before, so I guessed it was just nerves that had made me ill.

When we arrived at my cousin's apartment he introduced me to his wife and her daughter and the housekeeper that they had and then Adam and I rushed straight for the bathroom as we needed to bath asap.

Once we had freshened up my cousin took us to a restaurant in Wan Chai and we had a mixture of Chinese food which we all shared and then we went to a bar called Spicy Fingers and we sat outside drinking as it was so hot. It was so different being in Hong Kong as everywhere was busy all the time.

As we sat drinking people around us seemed friendly and there was no trouble from anyone, it was so nice to see everyone mixing in together.

We met one of my cousin's friends who was Chinese and he was a lovely friendly man and very clever and he sat and spoke with Adam and I for most of the evening.

When the night was over my cousin hailed a taxi down just like they do in New York and we went back to his apartment. Adam and I shared a room and we had bunkbeds, it was nice and cosy in there and I particularly liked the balcony that came off from the living room, as I could see all the buildings lit up at night time and it looked great.

The next day my cousin took us to a place called Stanley, it was a seaside town and it had a huge market there. As we travelled I started feeling sick again and my stomach felt real woozy, but I didn't say anything until we reached our destination and then I asked my cousin where the toilets were and I rushed inside and I was sick yet again, I couldn't understand it and it worried me a bit. But I wasn't going to let it spoil my holiday, as I'd waited for this for long enough.

We took some photographs outside a small temple and then we looked around the market, it was a lovely market and they sold lots of different things and everyone there was nice. Then we walked around and had some photographs taken with the sea behind us and when we faced the sea it was an amazing view, it looked just like something you'd see in a painting.

Later as it got to lunchtime we found a nice fish and chip shop and there was an old Chinese man walking around outside touting for business, he was very friendly and showed us to a table. It was extremely hot that day and my stomach still felt a bit dodgy, so I drank some water and then stood by a huge fan to try and cool down a bit. I guess I wasn't used to that kind of heat, but it was still lovely being in Hong Kong.

After we'd looked around a little longer we then made our way back to the car and back to my cousin's apartment and then a while later my cousin said he wanted to take my Son and I somewhere else to see. We then drove for a short distance and then got out of the car and as we walked along a pathway we suddenly had the best view I'd ever seen. We were high up on the Peak and we could see across Victoria Harbour to Kowloon. It was amazing and we walked from Hong Kong Island all the way around to Kowloon and back again. It was one of the best experiences I had in Hong Kong.

The next day my cousin had to work so we went out with his wife to Wan Chai and we went to a proper Chinese restaurant, nothing like a Chinese takeaway, this was like what you'd see in old movies. It had tables with white table cloths on and tiny cups that they kept refilling with tea every time they were empty and I tried lots of different food in there.

After we'd been there we met up with my cousin's step-daughter and she took Adam off with her to show him around and I went with my cousin's wife and had a face massage and facial cleansing. It was so relaxing and the lotions they used smelt lovely, it made me feel really refreshed.

Another day I looked around Wan Chai and they had lots of markets there, it was a bit smelly but that's because they sold lots of various kinds of fish.

Adam and I also had a massage and I had quite a petite lady do mine, but Adam had a butch lady and he suffered a bit of pain later that day, ha ha.

Another day we went to Hong Kong Central, it's very much like London with all the top named shops and then we walked to see Victoria Harbour close-up and we took a ferry to the other side of the harbour into Kowloon. Once there we went to the Avenue of Stars and there was a huge statue of Bruce Lee. I love Bruce Lee so I had to have a photograph next to him.

The view from there was just breath-taking, it was so much better than I'd imagined it to be.

I also met up with my cousin's children one evening as I'd never met them before and we had a nice meal out with them in Hong Kong Central.

One evening my cousin and his friends hired a boat and we went to a restaurant situated on the harbour, it was a fish restaurant. There were about nineteen of us and we sat around two large round tables. The waiters brought out all various kinds of fish and we took it in turns to help ourselves to the food. We had to turn the table so everyone had something to eat and I even ate with chop sticks. I tried Calamari which is squid in batter and it tasted quite nice, but I don't think I'd have tried it without batter because to look at part of a baby octopus wouldn't have looked very nice. I had crab and lobster and it was all delicious.

I had to use the ladies room whilst I was there and because it was such a big place I took the wrong turning coming back, I ended up in an area where there were two very old Chinese men sitting eating and they just stared at me, so I waved and said Hi and then quickly made my exit.

One day Adam and I boarded a train as we wanted to see the Tian Tan Buddha which was also known as the big buddha. It was in Ngong Ping, Lantau Island and to see it closely we had to go from the train onto a cable car. It was the scariest thing ever and it was extremely high, it was as high as the clouds and I screamed all the way to the top and what made it worse was me being clever I'd paid extra to have a glass floor, not a clever idea.

When we reached the top, there was a village with small shops, it was amazing, it was like another world seeing a village in the clouds.

We spent quite a few hours there and we could see the Tian Tan Buddha quite clearly, but to get even closer we had to climb lots of steps. I told Adam I didn't think I could manage to climb all those steps but he wasn't going to let me get out of it. As I climbed I thought I was going to die, not just because I was still out of breath, but because of the heat as well. But I'm glad I did it in the end because it was amazing to see the giant Buddha closely. As we made our way back down the steps I counted them and there were 230 steps, no wonder I thought I was going to die.

One evening we went to the Yacht Club and met up with my cousin's Chinese friend and the view from there was fantastic as it was night time and all the buildings were lit up.

Whilst I was in Hong Kong my cousin flew my Son and I out to the Philippines for four days and I saw real volcano's there which was something I'd never seen in real life only in pictures. My cousin showed me the rice fields that he had and there were lots and we had to walk quite a distance to see them all, but because it was hot I got tired quickly, so one of the workers there gave me a lift back to my cousin's house on his motorbike. I also went to see my cousin's ducks, there must have been over a thousand, but I had to wear a mask when I entered their pen because the smell was awful and there was a lot of dust from their poop. I collected eggs from them and put them in a basket, that was something I'd never done before and another time whilst I was in the Philippines I even held a baby goat and it was so cute.

Some of the local guys there took Adam and I out on a boat and it was great, it wasn't a huge boat it looked more like a rowing boat, but it did have an engine on it. I had a wonderful time that day and the guys were nice and friendly.

When we eventually got back to Hong Kong Adam and I started to find our way around and often went out on our own in the daytime. One day we went on the Big Bus Tour and that took us all around various parts of Hong Kong and we went to a place called Mongkok and I absolutely loved it there. To me that was how I'd imagined Hong Kong and China to be. It had lots of Chinese shops and signs lit up in Chinese writing and it was extremely busy, but I loved the hustle and bustle of the Chinese way of life. We went to a huge market there called Ladies market and we bought a few gifts for family and friends whilst we were there.

Before leaving Hong Kong I had to see the Peak once more and whilst I was there I also went into Madame Tussauds which was situated on the Peak. It had a lot of famous Chinese people in there, but also some famous

English and American people. I had a photograph taken with Muhammad Ali as he has always been my hero and with the Beatles.

I also took a trip on a boat to a place called Aberdeen, but we didn't get off the boat. We were given Chinese hats to put on to have photographs taken in and we had a floating restaurant in the background, it was the most beautiful looking restaurant I'd ever seen.

We met up with my cousin's children on several occasions and my cousin's son told Adam about a place he should take me to before we left Hong Kong, but my Son kept it a secret from me until we got there. We travelled by train and when we got off the train we crossed the road and walked up a steep hill. Then we had to climb lots of steps to visit a temple and 10,000 buddha's. As I struggled to climb the steps I realized I was climbing a mountain, but with steps, it was the hottest day since we'd been in Hong Kong so the heat was unbearable and my hair and clothes were soaked.

We could see the point of the roof of the temple in the distance, but I knew it was going to take us ages to reach the top. There were seats for people to take a break, but it was still challenging work trying to climb up something so high. When we reached the top, we realized we'd climbed up the wrong side of the mountain and we ended up in a monk's cemetery. We had to walk back down hundreds of steps and I was exhausted by then. I sat down and drank a cold can of coke and I even put the freezing can on my head, but the can got warm quite quickly as the heat from my head was so hot.

Once we were back at the bottom of the mountain Adam said let's climb the other side but I wasn't very enthusiastic, I was hot and tired and ready to give up, but he wouldn't let me. I once again climbed hundreds of steps, passing gold buddha statues as I climbed. They looked amazing and there were hundreds of them. I had to keep stopping as I climbed and quite a few times I really didn't think I was going to make it, but my Son wouldn't let me give up so I kept going and eventually reached the top. It was an amazing site seeing thousands of gold buddhas, ten thousand in all and I was glad that I'd seen them in the end, even though it almost killed me in the process.

I was so happy being out in Hong Kong and I'd forgot about all the tough times I'd had over the last few years. But my stomach still didn't feel right and late one night whilst at my cousin's I'd noticed on my underwear that I had spotted blood, but because I didn't have periods anymore I didn't have any sanitary towels, so I had to get one from my cousin's wife and it was all very embarrassing. I didn't bleed anymore whilst I was out in Hong Kong but I knew once I got back I had to mention it to my doctor.

On the last night of our holiday we went out with my cousin and we had a great night in Wan Chai, we drank beer and danced to a group that was playing and they were good. A lot of the groups that sing in Hong Kong are from the Philippines and they have amazing voices and sing all the latest songs that we know back in England.

On our last night I cried because I didn't want to leave Hong Kong, it had been an amazing holiday and I didn't want it to end. We'd been out there for three weeks but the time had gone so quick.

My cousin took us to the airport and we flew back to England, but I still wasn't happy about being back home. I wanted to see Todd of course but I also still wanted to be in Hong Kong.

When I got back home I'd now got the bug to travel and straight away I booked my next holiday with both my boys to take them to Rome for a week. I'd been through so much with being ill and being treated badly that I wanted to now enjoy my life and I didn't intend on wasting anymore of it.

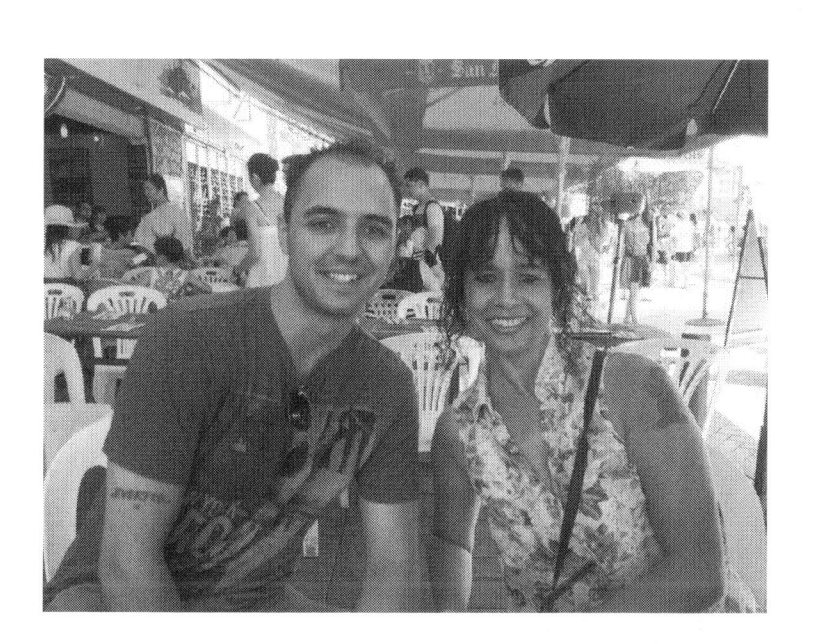

CHAPTER ELEVEN

After getting back from Hong Kong I was still buzzing and I couldn't wait to tell everyone about my experience. The only thing I wasn't looking forward to was the thought of going back to work. I hadn't been to work for a few months as I'd taken time of sick for depression and I still didn't want to go back there, but the summer holidays were now over so I had no choice.

I also made an appointment to see a doctor about the spotting I'd had whilst in Hong Kong, but when I saw the doctor it wasn't my usual one and after I explained to her what had happened to me, she didn't seem to think it was anything serious, so I left it at that.

It wasn't until a few months later when I made another appointment to see my usual doctor she said she'd read my notes and she wasn't happy leaving it, she seemed to think I needed to see a gynaecologist. A few weeks later I was sent to see a consultant in Canterbury and he examined me and after he told me *"We are looking for cancer"*, *"I said, yes, I guessed that"*, but I was thinking he could have worded it a bit better instead of just blurting out the C word.

He took a swab but then he told me I needed to have a biopsy taken and that I'd have to be put under anaesthetic at a later date. I then asked if I could possibly have the biopsy at Margate hospital rather than have to travel all the way to Canterbury again and he agreed. I felt sick as I'd been clear from breast cancer for quite a few years, but I was now worried that I could have cervical cancer, it was just awful.

I waited a few weeks for the appointment to arrive in the post and when it did my friend Kim said she'd come with me. She'd already been with me when I saw the consultant in Canterbury, so I thought it was nice of her to put herself out and come to the hospital with me again.

As I sat waiting with other patients in the waiting room I just wanted to go home. I was scared at the thought of what they'd find, but even after having a biopsy I still wouldn't know the results straight away.

I was at the hospital about 7.30 am but I didn't get called down to theatre until about 3pm and the wait was just draining.

As I lay on the bed the nurses seemed nice and friendly and then the anaesthetist came into the room and explained to me what he'd be doing, but I knew exactly how anaesthetic worked after all I'd had plenty of operations before.

I don't remember much just that the needle went into my hand and I started going fuzzy headed. When I woke up I couldn't move I was wrapped up like a mummy and even had blankets around my head. As I looked around the nurse came over to me and said that whilst I was under anaesthetic my temperature dropped a lot and they had to wrap me up to keep me warm as they were quite worried. Nothing ever seemed to go straight forward where I was concerned, but at least I'd had the biopsy done and hopefully I could soon go home.

The nurse left me for a while and then made me a hot drink, but I was only allowed to take small sips not big mouthfuls in case it made me sick. Luckily I wasn't sick this time I actually felt fine, so a few hours later I was allowed home. But even though I only lived about a ten-minute walk from the hospital I decided to get a taxi home, as I didn't want to walk half way home and collapse. My friend stayed the night at my house that night which was nice of her, but I felt fine, it was just another day at the hospital for me, ha ha.

I took the next day off work as I wasn't supposed to do anything for three days and as it was Friday by then it worked out fine, as I then had the weekend to rest as well. My friend stayed with me over the weekend as she didn't have any commitments, she was single just like me and her daughter was grown up.

I sometimes went out with her on a Saturday night but only now and again, I didn't go out every week, but my friend went out a lot more with ladies that she knew. When I did go out we'd got to Ramsgate seafront and drink in the bars down there and then we'd end up in a bar called the Jazz Room that stayed open late. One day whilst I was in there a guy said hello to my friend, I didn't know him but I recognized him from somewhere but I couldn't remember where. I asked my friend who he was and she said, *"he always comes down here"*. I kept looking at him but I still couldn't remember where I'd seen him and it wasn't until a few months later I got talking to him one night and for some strange reason he brought up that he used to have a motorbike and then it dawned on me where I'd seen him. When I was two my parents moved to a cul-de-sac and that's where I recognized this guy from. He didn't live in the same street but when I was about ten he dated a girl who lived a few doors away from me and when I mentioned it to him he admitted he was that guy. I couldn't believe that I'd remembered him after all those years and I was only ten then and he was about seventeen. But I remember him having a motorbike because he parked it outside the house on the road and my Sister dared me to climb onto it one day and as I did he came out of the house and told me off. When I told him he laughed, and he said he would have told anyone off for touching his motorbike as that was his pride and joy. Thinking about it now I didn't blame him.

Whenever I went out and I used to see that guy I'd always speak to him and I did quite like him, but I hadn't long had my divorce so I wasn't really looking for a relationship at that time.

About a week after having my biopsy I had a letter come through the post, it was my results and when I opened it my heart raced, but I'd got the all clear, I hadn't got cervical cancer after all, but I still don't know why I had a spotting of blood unless it was to do with the pressure of flying to Hong Kong.

I went back to work and told everyone my good news and the people there were really pleased for me.

I was still looking for another job but I didn't find it very easy finding anything else, so I just had to stick with the job I had.

A few months after having my biopsy I flew to Rome with my two Sons, my friend looked after my house and dog for me, but I was only going for a week this time, not three weeks like last time.

When we arrived in Rome we were told we couldn't land at that airport as they'd been an incident there, so we had to fly further and land at army type airport, but we weren't allowed off the plane we had to wait until the pilot was given the go-ahead to fly back to Rome. By the time we arrived in Rome it was late and we'd missed our taxi ride that was supposed to take us to our hotel, so we had to pay again for another taxi to take us.

I was a bit scared when we got into this guy's car as the doors locked and he looked rather scary and as he drove he didn't speak to us, he seemed quite serious. I whispered to my Son's that we could be being taken somewhere by gangsters for all we know, as we didn't know who this guy was. They looked at me and laughed but I must admit I was quite scared, or maybe my over thinking was scaring me more.

We arrived at the hotel about 1am and by then we were all shattered, so once we were shown to our rooms we went straight to bed.

The next day we had breakfast at the hotel as that was included in the price and it was lovely, there was so much food to choose from. We then went out and viewed museums and churches that day and luckily the weather stayed nice because we had to walk quite a distance from our hotel. I suppose we could have taken a train but I like to view all the areas as I walk.

As we walked along the streets we soon noticed how dangerous people drove, they didn't slow down when we crossed the road and even on a zebra crossing they didn't stop, we'd had to just run and hope we didn't get knocked down.

As we looked at churches they were nothing like we have in England, every church in Rome was decorated with art, there were drawings of paintings everywhere from walls to ceiling and it looked amazing.

I'm not an over religious person but I do have my own beliefs, but I'm not Catholic like most of the people in Rome, my religion is Church of England.

But I had always admired Pope John Paul 11 I thought he was an amazing man and he gave so much hope and joy to the entire world. I remember watching him on TV standing on the balcony of the Vatican on Easter Sunday and I loved seeing the crowds just looking at him in amazement as they stood in St Peter's Square. I always said I'd love to stand in that square one day and look up at the Vatican and I finally got my wish. I went to the Vatican and I stood in St Peter's Square and looked up at the Vatican, but the Pope wasn't there that day, but I didn't mind as I'd still done what I'd set out to do. The Vatican is a beautiful building and when I went inside I prayed that everyone would be free from cancer, including myself. I just hope my prayers are answered very soon and everyone is free from this horrible disease.

Next door to the Vatican is the Sistine Chapel and as I walked inside there were paintings everywhere and it was the most amazing place I'd ever seen, it was beautiful and if any of you people that are reading this book have never seen it, I advise you to go there as you won't be disappointed.

Every day that I was in Rome we went somewhere different and every place I went to was amazing. People kneeled praying and I could see how deeply they felt about their religion, it was quite moving.

I went to see the Colosseum one day and as I stood in a queue waiting to go in it was quite cold in there. It was very big and as I walked around I found a piece of concrete which had come away from the Colosseum wall, so I picked it up and put it in my pocket, so now I have part of the Colosseum with me in my home.

About a mile from the Colosseum we went to a place that had steps inside, they were called Jesus steps and these steps are reported to be the steps that Jesus climbed just before he was crucified, they had been moved from Jerusalem.

They are marble steps covered with wood. There are glass enclosed port holes where Jesus blood had been spilled and when you walk the 28 steps you must crawl up them on your knees. It was very emotional watching people do this and kissing the stairs as they climbed.

I went all over Rome whilst I was there and I viewed some amazing buildings, but the only one I didn't get to see was the Trevi Fountain, as when we got there it had scaffolding all around it as it was being repaired.

I'm so glad I went to Rome and took both my Son's with me, it was the first holiday we'd ever had together as a family. A few years before that I would never have dreamt I'd be on holiday with both my boys, it's surprising how quick someone's life can change.

My friend Kim who I'd known since I was eleven had been good to me helping look after my dog whilst I was away and yet she was suffering with health problems herself. She had torn tendons in her foot and some days she could hardly walk it was that painful. She was due to go into hospital to have it operated on, so I said once the operation was over she could stay at my house to recuperate. She'd have been on her own if I hadn't of helped her and I wasn't going to let that happen as she'd done a lot for me and even came to visit me in Cambridgeshire just after I had finished my treatment.

I went with her to the hospital and luckily it was at Margate so it wasn't far from where I lived. I stayed with her all day and was waiting for her when she came out from theatre and she seemed fine. Her foot was bandaged up and she wasn't allowed to walk on it, so they gave her a Zimmer frame to use to help her walk. I helped as much as I could and helped her wash etc. as it was hard for her to balance herself and I cooked her meals whilst she was with me. She stayed with me just over a week and once she was well we planned to go out and celebrate.

It took quite a few weeks for Kim's foot to heal, but even after the operation she still had some pain, but she was told there was nothing more they could do.

Once she was well enough we had a night out and I danced all night, I loved dancing and I danced all around the dance floor like a loon ha ha. I wasn't interested in going out and meeting guys, I just loved going out to listen to the music that I liked and just generally having an enjoyable time.

I knew some of Kim's friends by now and I still sometimes saw the guy who's motorbike I climbed on as a child. We often had a chat and sometimes at the end of the night we'd walk up to the chip shop with him and buy a bag of chips and then share a taxi home.

I was still working at the school but I hated every minute of it, but the lady boss that I had who I didn't like very much was fine with me now, ever since I'd had time off with depression and complained about my work load she spoke to me civil, so maybe by me speaking up and fighting for my rights did the trick.

By this time not only had Sonia and my lead cleaner left, but I'd now also lost my friend Carlene as well, as she'd also left the school, so I wasn't enjoying the job at all.

I applied for lots of jobs but I wasn't hearing anything back and it was getting me down.

One day as I was looking through the local paper I saw an advertisement that said that Gerry and the Pacemakers were coming to Margate, I was jumping around the room as I'd been brought up with rock 'n' roll music and 60's music and I loved it and my Sister and I had always loved Gerry Marsden as a child and we both always wanted to see him. I phoned my Sister straight away and told her that we had to go and she was excited as much as I was, so I booked two tickets as soon as I got off the phone from speaking with my her. It seemed that finally I was doing something with my life, I was having holidays, going out when I wanted and just living my life again and I was happy and I didn't need a guy in my life to enjoy myself, I was quite happy the way I was being single.

A few weeks before I was due to see Gerry and the Pacemakers I finally had an interview for another job and this time it wasn't to do cleaning, it was to work in a pie shop in Margate and it was only about a five-minute walk from where I lived. I went and spoke with the manager and the interview went well, but he had other people to see so I just had to keep my fingers crossed. But a few days later the manager of the shop phoned me and he told me I'd got the job, I was so happy I was finally getting out of a job I hated and I felt great.

A few days before starting my new job I went to see Gerry and the Pacemakers and they were amazing. My Sister and I were the youngest people in the theatre and we had lots of older people say to us that we were too young to remember Gerry Marsden. But I told them that our parents had liked their music, so we knew all their songs at an early age. We had a great night and I was so glad I'd seen him, it had been one of my ambitions to one day see Gerry and the Pacemakers.

Everything seemed to be going well for me now and I was really enjoying my life.

When I started work at the pie shop I had to cook all the food such as, sausage rolls, meat pies, fruit pies, chicken, sausages, hot dogs etc. and I also served customers. I loved it and although it was a job I enjoyed it.

I was also working more hours so I had more money and I decided to book another holiday but for the next year. I decided to go back to Hong Kong and take my youngest

Son Todd with me this time, as he didn't get to go the last time I went. But instead of staying with my cousin this time I booked us into a hotel, I didn't want to be a burden to my cousin, after all he'd already been good to me letting me stay at his apartment for three weeks before.

I had a long wait to go before my holiday as I had almost a year to go, but it gave me something to look forward too. I worked every day but had weekends off which was good and the guys I worked with were nice. Most of them were younger than me but I got on with people of all ages. I even got on great with customers of all ages and it didn't take me long to get to know my regulars. I had guys who worked on building sites come into our shop, they'd be a bit cheeky and make me laugh, but I gave as good as I got. Most of the workman were about my Sons age but they were a good bunch of guys. I even had older people stand chatting with me and I think it broke up their day, but I didn't mind. I had a few favourite customers and one was an older guy, he would always come in for a bacon roll and he'd give me a lot of stick, but it was all in wholesome fun. I remember one day I had to lift a glass door upwards to clean one of the food heater units, but I used to hold it as I cleaned in case it fell on me. But I was told that it stayed up on its own, so one day I let it go and cleaned it, but it slowly came down on the back of my neck. I fell forward into the unit and a customer who was standing next to me just watched, he didn't even help me. I managed to lift the glass door up and get out but it had hurt my neck. I told one of the ladies there what happened and she looked at my neck and said I had a line going across it where the glass had hit me. She then went out the back and watched it back on camera and I don't think I've ever heard anyone laugh so much in my life, she couldn't stop she thought it was hilarious. But looking at it myself I could see the funny side, but what I didn't understand was why the customer stood and watched it happen, I could have lost my head ha ha.

I knew lots of people in Margate and with Dreamland reopening soon it gave us a lot more trade, the builders working at Dreamland always came to us for food and when it opened we were even given discount tickets on entry.

Margate has changed quite a lot since I was a child, people seem to go abroad now rather than come to seaside towns. But I still like sitting down by the beach on the white steps, just watching everyone go by and looking at the sea.

When I was a girl I used to love Dreamland and I loved the rides especially the scenic railway as that was the main attraction and probably still is.

How times change from when you're small you don't think anything bad can happen at that age and I'd have never have dreamt that I'd one day have breast cancer and would have to have Chemotherapy, you just don't know what the future holds.

That is why once I got better and moved back to Kent I wasn't going to waste anymore of my life, I'd been stuck in a village and felt trapped for way to long and now I had a fresh start and I was enjoying every minute of it.

As for my ex-husband I hardly even thought of him anymore, but he did phone me on the odd occasion and I was civil to him, after all we were friend's now nothing more.

CHAPTER TWELVE

I had now stopped going to the hospital for regular check-ups, but I still had to have mammograms every two years, unless of course anything was wrong then I would have to see my doctor straight away.

I was still on Tamoxifen as I must take them until 2020 but taking one tablet a day wasn't that bad, I just set an alarm on my mobile to remind me.

As I had a bit more money now I went out on a Saturday night at least twice a month instead of just the once. I loved getting out as when my children were small I never got the chance, but now I was out with girl-friends and having a wonderful time every other week.

Todd was now at college and he had his own friends he went out with and the same with my eldest Son Adam.

But even though I was enjoying myself at last, cancer was never far from my mind, it never really leaves you once you've had it. I always felt myself just in case anymore lumps appeared, but even feeling the slightest bump makes you panic even if you know it's nothing really. The trouble is I have lots of lumps on my arms and even one on my hip, but I was told that they're nothing to worry about as its normal. But I never had them as a child so why did I have them now?

My thyroid was now a lot better and I didn't take tablets for that anymore and luckily, I hadn't relapsed, but I did still have regular blood tests and sometimes I had to take Folic Acid tablets as I was still out of breath, as I was obviously lacking in certain vitamins.

I was eating healthier though and I could take food home from the pie shop that I worked in, if there was anything left at the end of the day. That helped me out a bit because

I didn't always feel like cooking once I'd got home after I'd done a whole day's work.

A lot of the shops had closed in Margate but we seemed quite busy in our shop, but it was getting worrying, as all the big shops were moving out of town up to Westwood Cross. I didn't want to lose my job again as it had taken me ages to get back into retail and I was soon to be going back to Hong Kong for two and a half weeks, so I needed every penny I could get.

I'd saved hard for this holiday but I had promised Todd I'd take him to Hong Kong so I wasn't going to let him down. It was hot in England now and it felt quite unbearable working in the shop, I did all the cooking so I got extremely hot, but in the winter it was freezing in the shop and having to get food from the walk-in freezer was horrible as it was so cold and it took ages to warm up again after. But I'd rather be hot than cold and I was looking forward to travelling to Hong Kong again and although it was their rainy season, it was still very humid there.

I had already warned Todd about when we get outside to expect to feel the heat on you straight away and as we arrived in Hong Kong and walked outside the airport he soon knew what I meant and as he felt the heat he looked at me and smiled. We got a taxi to our hotel which took about a forty-five-minute journey and as the taxi driver drove I pointed to some of the building and told Todd which one my cousin worked in. Todd was amazed by the stunning buildings as I knew he would be, but that was just the beginning of our holiday, I had so much more to show him.

The hotel was nice and clean but the rooms weren't huge, they were quite cosy really and we had a view looking over a cemetery, but I didn't mind because we were going to be out most of the time and only come back to the hotel to sleep.

We didn't go out anywhere the first night as we were so tired, we just both had a bath and went to bed. The next day we went to Causeway Bay as I hadn't been there the last time I went to Hong Kong, so it was nice to go somewhere different. There were lots of shops to view and although it wasn't the best place in Hong Kong it was still nice to view a different part of the country. I took Todd to other places I'd already seen before such as Hong Kong Central where all the top named shops were and Todd somehow found a Michael Jordan shop that he liked. The hotel was situated in Wan Chai so we didn't have to far to walk to various parts of that town and bus stops were right outside our hotel.

We found a nice restaurant in Wan Chai and we had a lovely Carbonara there and other days we tried quite a few of the Chinese restaurants nearby.

I hadn't felt ill this time after I'd travelled and I still don't know why I was sick before or why I spotted last time I was there.

I took Todd to Stanley one day and he saw the market I'd told him about and about the lovely fish and chip shop that was there. I also met up with my cousin and he drove us to a place called Repulse Bay and it was hot that day. I took my flipflops off to walk on the beach, but I soon put them back on again as the sand was boiling hot.

Another day I took Todd to Ocean Park as it had a fairground there and a zoo and we sat and watched the dolphin display whilst we were there which was lovely. I also met up with my cousins Son and daughter and we went out for dinner with them on several evenings.

I loved Mongkok when I was there before so I had to show Todd that place, we got a big bus tour that took us there and Todd absolutely loved the market they had there and whilst in Hong Kong Central another day, we went on the Ferris wheel and we could see for miles all around Hong Kong.

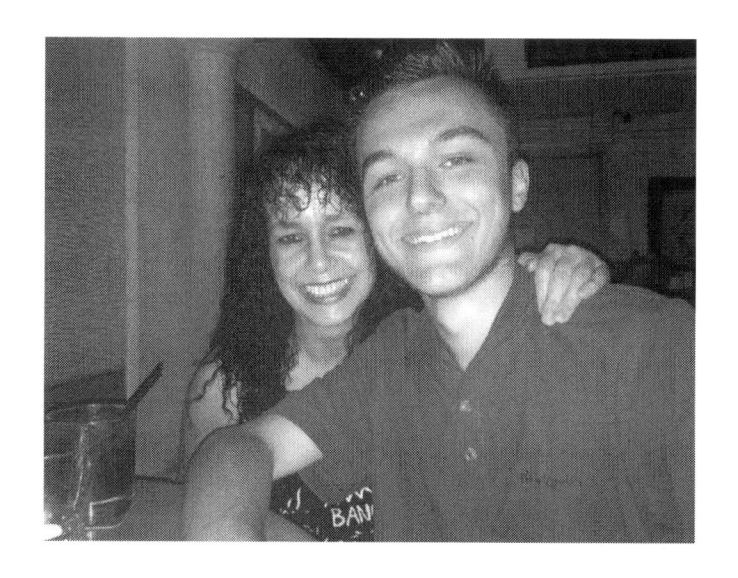

I never would have dreamt a few years before I would go to Hong Kong once let alone twice, I couldn't believe how much my life had changed since I'd been ill.
But I knew I wouldn't get another holiday for a while as travelling to Hong Kong had cost a lot of money, so once I was home I decided that if I travelled anywhere it would be in the United kingdom.
After being back from Hong Kong about two months I one day found another lump in my breast, it was the left breast the same one as before. I showed my Sister where the lump was and she seemed to think as it was near the scar that I had on my breast from where I'd had the tumour removed, that it could possibly be just scar tissue. But I still went to my doctors and I was referred to the hospital for a mammogram. I had the mammogram and I had to wait for the result, but it wasn't conclusive enough, so I had to have an Ultra Sound Scan and that showed that it

was scar tissue. I was so relieved because after last time when I was ill you always seem to expect the worst, but on this occasion I was fine.

I went up to London that weekend and I travelled around Westminster and it was lovely, I think people sometimes forget how lovely our country is here in the UK and yet we have some beautiful places to visit.

I went to Harwich Park first and fed the squirrels and I even had a blue tit land on my hand and I saw a fox close and he was beautiful. The squirrels were funny because they'd take the nuts from you and one squirrel even held my finger as he took a nut and another ran up my friend's leg and quickly took a nut from their hand, it was very funny to watch. It's a lovely park and once you're on top of the hill you have a pleasant view.

I went for breakfast in the Cutty Sark Café which wasn't far from where the actual Cutty Sark ship is situated, I remember going on that ship when I was a child, I went with the school. The Café did a lovely full English breakfast and I've been back there a few times.

I also went to Camden in the evening to the World's End pub and that was different to what I expected, it was quite big and had different floor levels you could go on. It was nice just to get away from everything and for a while I didn't even think about cancer.

But then one day I had a hospital appointment come through the post, it was for a check-up for the scar tissue lump I'd found a few months before. The consultant I had was nice and she spoke to me as she examined me, but she suddenly found another lump in the middle of my breast this time and it wasn't there the last time she had checked me, even I'd missed this lump.

She told me she'd have to book me in for a mammogram and I thought she meant for that day, but she then told me she couldn't do it that day they'd have to send an appointment out to me. I left the hospital feeling numb as it had only been a few months since the last cancer scare, I couldn't take much more and I felt sick.

Everyone told me not to worry but when you find a lump you can't help but worry, especially when you've had breast cancer before.

My Sister again said to me it's probably scar tissue, but this lump was in the middle of my breast, it was nowhere near the scar that I had. I was really worried this time and I couldn't sleep and I felt like it was history repeating itself all over again. To make things even worse was that I'd waited over a week for an appointment for a mammogram, but in the end, I couldn't wait any longer so I phoned the hospital. I explained to my consultant's secretary about the lump and that I'd had breast cancer before, but she told me I'd have to wait over a month for an appointment. I couldn't believe what I was hearing, I was panicking now because I needed to know the result, but having to wait another month was just ridiculous. I wasn't happy and I started phoning the hospital every day, I just wanted to have a mammogram not an operation, so surely, they could book me in. But the secretary was still adamant I'd have to wait a month, but I wasn't going to give up easily, so she said she'd have a word with my consultant, but even she said no I'd have to wait. I couldn't believe it as when I was at Addenbrooke's hospital they done everything so quickly, they were amazing.

I was up all night not being able to sleep the waiting was terrible. But out of the blue I got a phone call to say they could give me an earlier appointment and I jumped at the chance to have the mammogram. A few days later I went to the hospital and had the mammogram but again it was inconclusive, so I had to have another Ultra Sound Scan, but even that couldn't tell them whether it was cancer or not. I had to have a biopsy taken and then I had to wait a week or so for the result, it was just awful. I left the hospital thinking the worst because of where it was on my breast and it felt quite big.

That week leading up to getting my results seemed a lifetime away and when I did finally arrive at the hospital I was petrified. I was thinking I could be starting treatment all over again, but what if this time it didn't work.

I sat in the waiting room fidgeting and fiddling with my fingers, it was just nerves I guess. But the wait is just the worst feeling ever, as it gives you time to think and I do a lot of that and maybe I over think things as well.

Once I was called into the consulting room I was asked to lay on a bed so I could be examined, I then lay waiting for the doctor to come into the room. As she examined me she asked me questions about my previous lumps in my breast and then she said she had to go and get my notes, so I still wasn't told my biopsy results straight away. When she came back into the room she then told me the lump in my breast was nothing to worry about, it was just fibrous tissue. I was so relieved and I couldn't wait to get out of the hospital and tell everyone I knew that I was fine.

It's such a scary feeling when you find a lump and it's even worse when you've already had breast cancer before, because any lump you find you always think, has it come back again.

As I walked home from the hospital everything felt different, I was so happy and nothing was going to destroy my day. A huge weight had been lifted from me and the feeling I had inside felt wonderful.

I went home and went straight on Facebook to let everyone know that I was fine and I had lots of replies from friends congratulating me and it was nice to read their comments, having that support from people makes an enormous difference in someone's life.

I've since joined breast cancer groups on Facebook and I sometimes comment on what people write as they go through their treatment. I like to wish people well as it gives them a boost to know there are people out there that care.

Anyone that goes through any type of cancer needs all the support they can get, it was talking to people on Facebook that got me through the dark times when I was ill.

Many times I could have just given up because I didn't have the support from my husband, but I fought it because I wanted to live and I have two beautiful Sons who need me.

I have now been cancer free for seven years and although I'm clear that doesn't mean I don't think about it. Having cancer never really leaves you and any slight illness makes you worry that you've got cancer back again. It's a horrible feeling and anyone that's had cancer would probably agree with what I'm saying.

My Aunt recently passed away from cancer but whilst she was ill she confided in me quite a lot. She'd ask me questions about cancer and the treatment and if I had an answer I would try and explain things to her as best I could without frightening her. When my Aunt had Chemotherapy, she phoned me and said that she didn't realize what I'd gone through, but now she was in that situation she understood how awful the treatment is.

Because my Aunt lived away from me in Essex we didn't get to see each other every day, but I remember I went to see her on her last birthday. I didn't tell her I was coming to Essex I just turned up at my cousin's house where my Aunt was staying and I walked into the living room where my Aunt was sitting in a chair. She couldn't see my face because I had a few balloons in front of my face, but then I moved them away and said Happy Birthday. It was lovely seeing the surprised look upon her face and I'll never forget that day and I'm so glad I went to see her on her birthday as that was her last birthday and the last time I got to see her.

The little things people do to make you feel special when you're ill make such a difference and it does boost you up immensely.

I remember sending my Aunt flowers when she had her first three courses of Chemotherapy, I'd send them a few days after she'd had her treatment as I knew it would boost her up on her ill time. She also kept a teddy bear that I'd bought her when she was in hospital and she called it her lucky bear and once she was out of hospital she kept the teddy beside the chair she sat in at her house.

It's just little things like that that make such a difference, you don't have to spend thousands of pounds to make someone happy, even by sending a card is greatly received. With me talking to people on Facebook got me through my day, but without my friends and family to talk to I don't know how I would have coped. Talking about my illness was the best remedy for me, it helped me get through all the tough times.

Since being back in Kent with my family and friends I haven't been happier, but I do still have bad days when I worry about my health, but I'm one of the lucky ones I'm alive. We all have worries in our lives about money etc, but if you've got good health you should always think yourselves lucky and try and live life to the full.

I try to make the most of everyday now that I'm well and when the weather is nice I try and get out as much as I can. I'm not a wintry weather person I hibernate in the Winter, but I love the Summer and getting out to watch functions in the area, especially on bank holidays as that brings hundreds of local people together.

I also like writing and when my children were small I used to write short stories to read to them before bedtime, but now that they're older I obviously can't write for them anymore. But a few months ago, I had an idea, as I like writing so much I thought I'd write some more children's stories and put them on Amazon, that way a wider audience gets to read them. One of my stories is called Escape to Goblin City and the other is called Gideon the Laziest Leprechaun. I have them on Amazon books selling in book form or on Amazon Kindle. I've also written some more books for adults. A Father's Disapproval, The Lady of Beaufort Manor and a 50's story called Motorbikes and Party Lights. The adult ones are soon to be put on Amazon I'm just waiting for the covers to be finished, but please look out for them.

By writing these stories gave me an idea to write a book about my experience with breast cancer, as I thought if I sold any I could give some of the royalties to Breast Cancer Research, that way I would be giving something back and I would hopefully be helping others on their road to recovery.

I just wanted to let people know that there is life after breast cancer and although at the time of going through all the horrible treatment you can't see an end to it, there is hope and a lot more out there for you to live a normal life again.

Don't give up the fight no matter how awful the treatment is because that won't last forever, just keep thinking life will get better and if you do lose your hair it's not the end of the world it will grow back again.

I'm quite a strong-minded person but there were times when I thought I can't do this anymore, but I think a lot of that was not having the support I needed from my husband, that is why once I was stronger I made him move out because I felt that he had broken his marriage vows, the part that says in sickness and in health. But not everyone goes through what I went through, as most loyal husbands or partners are supportive and will help you through the bad days.

I'm still single and I'm not looking for a partner, I'm happy as I am. I'm not saying I'll always be on my own, but for the time being I'm enjoying just being alive and I'm enjoying writing my books.

For anyone who is going through breast cancer or any other type of cancer, I would like to wish you all well and maybe one day like me you can write about your experience to give others hope and although this is the end of my story, the next chapter in my life is about to begin and I'm going to enjoy every moment of it.

THE END

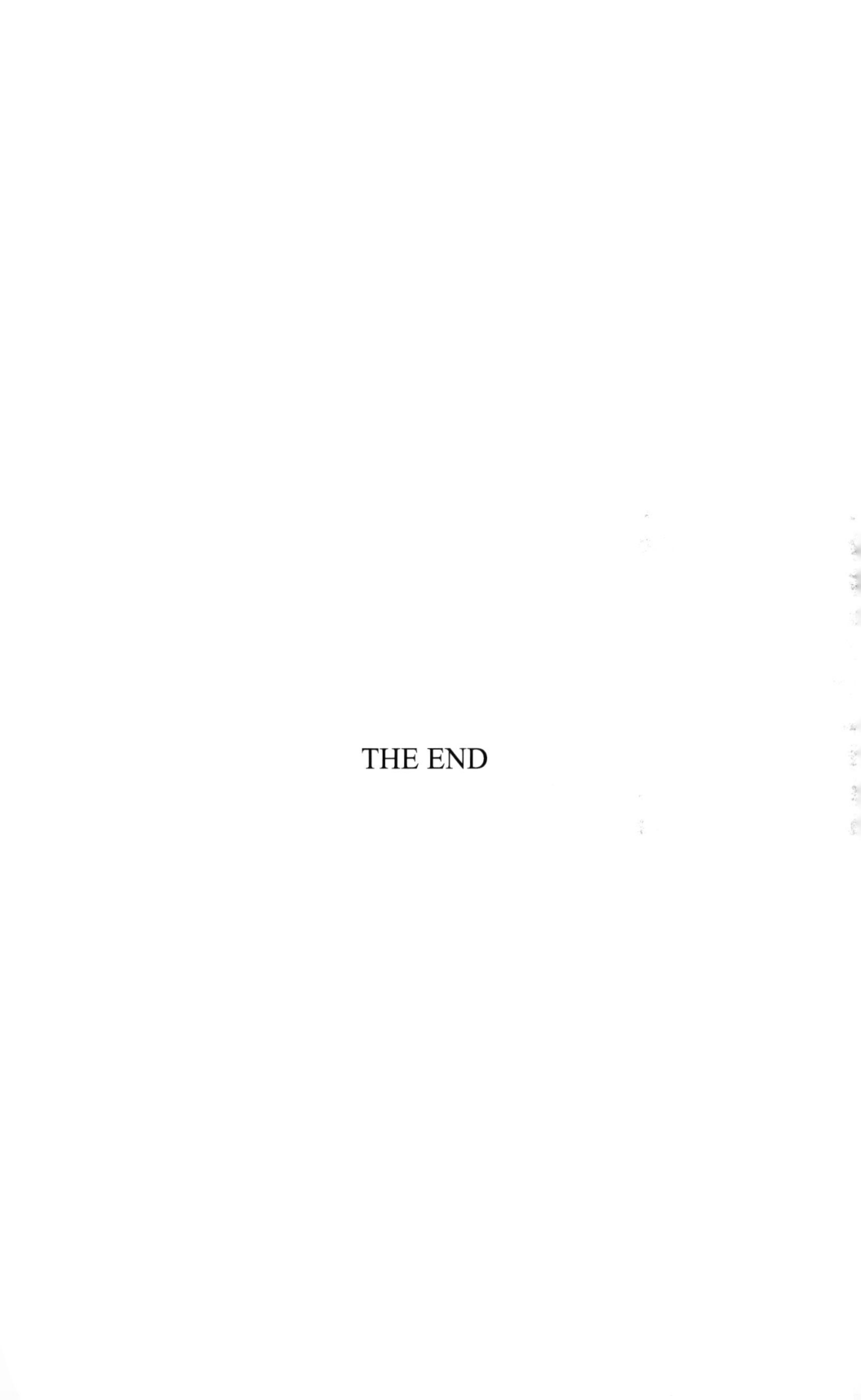

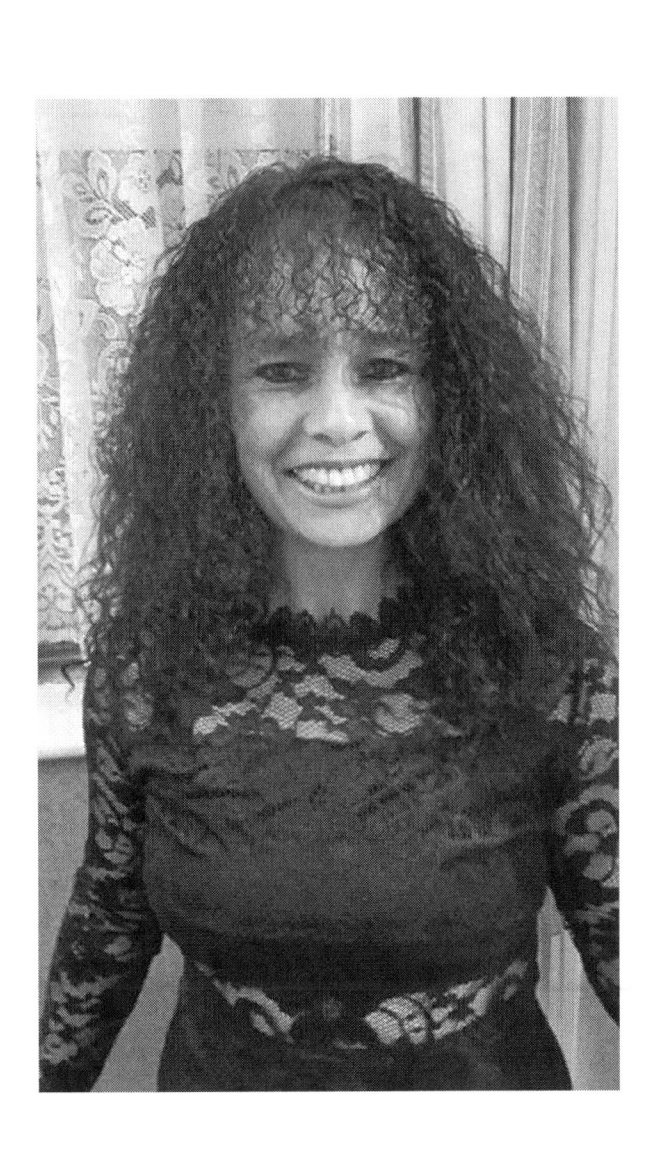

Printed in Great Britain
by Amazon